ENOUGH
ALREADY!

A GUIDE TO RECOVERY FROM ALCOHOL AND DRUG ADDICTION

BOB TYLER, BA, CADC II, ICADC

FOREWORD BY TERENCE GORSKI

Outskirts Press, Inc.
Denver, Colorado

Enough Already!
A Guide to Recovery from Alcohol and Drug Addiction

Outskirts Press
http://www.outskirtspress.com

ISBN-10: 1-59800-213-9
ISBN-13: 978-1-59800-213-3

Cover image by Tony Chavez Design

Image is symbolic of the dark hole alcoholics and addicts dig for themselves through their continued use. When a person has had *"Enough Already!"*, the path of recovery is the 12 steps, which lead from darkness to light."

Outskirts Press and the "OP" logo are trademarks belonging to Outskirts Press, Inc.

Printed in the United States of America

AUTHOR'S NOTE

The purpose of this book is to provide information in regard to the subject matter covered. It is meant for educational and entertainment purposes. It is not intended to render medical advice, therapy, or other professional services. Such professional services should be sought out if needed. The author and Humble House Publishing shall have neither liability nor responsibility to any person or entity with respect to any loss or damage caused, or alleged to be caused, directly or indirectly by the information contained in this book. If you wish not to be bound by this disclaimer, please return the book for a refund.

CONTENTS

ACKNOWLEDGEMENTS

I first want to thank my very knowledgeable and skilled friends who took the time to edit and critique this book: Robin Tyler (my wife), Rowdy Yates, Linda White, Terri Melvin, Terence Brown, Lori Phelps, Rhonda Messamore', Michael Axelrod, Mary Rowland (my mom), Larry Oliff, Dee O'Dell, Peter Agnew, John Moore, Colleen Ecker, Christina Sweet, Bradley Smith, and Chris Kaspar for his technical assistance.

I also want to acknowledge: the patients and colleagues I've worked with over the years who taught me the information in this book; Pastor O.K. Anderson whose love and guidance helped Robin and I to keep things in perspective, reminded us of God's unconditional love, and referred us to people who helped us change our lives; Jim Fulton, Mary Catherine Fitzgerald, Kay Poggi, Jane Meade, Larry Lakeshore, Bill Cullen, and Daniel Gatlin – the incredible counseling team which helped me get my life back; Michael Alvarez, a skilled therapist whose interventions aided my continued growth in recovery and which I continue to pass on to other recovering people; David Lisonbee of Twin Town Treatment Centers, my current employer and friend, who has taught me how to be a good boss and whose confidence in me has significantly facilitated my growth in this profession; Bob S., my current sponsor, who is always there when I need him; and my sober support system, including my brother Ken, who picks me up when I'm down, and who keeps me humble and grateful when I'm up.

I owe a special debt of gratitude to: my mother, Mary Rowland, who has always given me the love, understanding, and confidence I've needed to get through very difficult times and through life in general; my father, Ellis Tyler, who showed me the importance of honesty, integrity, and what a hard days work looks like; and both my parents who managed to raise me and my siblings, Mike, Dave, Ken, and Robin, in a way that makes them the finest and most respectable people I know; Robin, my lovely bride, who encouraged and gave me the confidence to write this book, who walked with me through the peaks and valleys, and who continues to love me unconditionally; and Christopher, Daniel, Timothy, and Cali, my children who, along with Robin, are the loves of my life and who are at the top of my gratitude list. I am very blessed!

FOREWORD

Enough Already is the story of one man's immersion in the program of recovery. From addict to counselor, Bob Tyler invites us to share his journey and gives clear suggestions as to what will work, if we work them. Bob reminds us that recovery can be elusive and how information and a structured program are essential to creating a clean and sober life that provide the miracle that recovering people seek.

Alcoholism and drug abuse are substance use disorders that result from the use of mind-altering substances by people who have biopsychosocial (physical, psychological, and social) risk factors that positively reinforce continued use of mind-altering substances and negatively reinforce abstinence.

An effective program of recovery will be based upon access to treatment, dignity and respect for the individual, and a continuum of care that meets the emerging needs of the recovering person. The most appropriate goal for the treatment of substance dependence is the development of a personally meaningful lifestyle that involves productive functioning in the family, workplace, and society.

The first step to recovery is abstinence from alcohol and other mind-altering drugs. Bob Tyler shares his personal experience of choosing abstinence and the consequences of his addictive lifestyle.

The second step is the development of a structured recovery program that supports abstinence and the development of a lifestyle centered around sober and responsible activities. The 12 Step programs are the most accessible recovery programs available and can work as Bob has outlined in *Enough Already.*

The third step is to both understand and begin the repair of the biopsychosocial (physical, psychological, and social) damage caused by the substance use disorders. And the final step is to develop positive personality and lifestyle changes that support continued abstinence.

Bob understands addiction and shares with you how to embrace recovery and work the 12 Step program of your choice. *Enough Already* provides numerous suggestions for designing a recovery program that fit the unique needs of each person pursuing recovery. Bob clearly outlines the path you will walk and gives personal examples of how he overcame many of the obstacles to recovery success.

Enough Already is an easy read, packed with emotion and valuable information. Read what Bob has written, try it out in your own life, and you will experience what recovery can do for you.

Terence T. Gorski
President and Founder
CENAPS Corporation

Dedicated to the memory of my friend and mentor, James Fulton Jr., a man whose caring and wisdom changed the course of my life…

…and Rowdy Yates, a friend and peer, who dedicated his life to helping alcoholics and addicts to recover.

INTRODUCTION

Having just finished smoking a joint in my car outside of the front entrance at work, I made a decision: "I really think I'm going to quit drugs and alcohol for good." After all, my wife and I were purchasing our first home and had gone for the final walk-through the previous day (Robin had somehow managed to save enough money for the down payment despite the thousands I spent on drugs in my using career). I wanted to get a fresh start in our new home and put all of the negative consequences of a drug and alcohol-filled life behind me. As I put out a cigarette, I thought, "Maybe I'll even quit these things too." I decided I would call Robin to let her know of all these noble thoughts I'd been having. I stepped back into the print shop my father owned and, with great excitement and anticipation, dialed the number for home. I knew she would share my excitement, since our lives would now be changing just as we were buying our long awaited first home.

My heart was pounding as I dialed the number and it began to ring. Robin answered the phone and, with much enthusiasm, I started into the dreams I had for our new life. I was very proud of myself as I spoke the words, "Robin, I have finally decided that I am going to quit drugs and alcohol once and for all." She suddenly interrupted me with words that pierced my heart, "Bob, my bags are packed and I'm leaving you." I was in utter shock! Had she not heard what I was saying? I was finally going to change my ways. I promptly told her something like, "Wait a minute – let's talk about this." She interrupted me again and stated she had put a lot of thought into this and was going through with it. She had heard such promises before and, after short periods of sobriety, was always disappointed by the resumption of my use. She continued by stating she loved me, but could not go on living like this anymore. I responded by telling her I was coming home right away and if she truly loved me, she would be there and we could talk about this. I promptly hung up the phone with the confidence I had struck a chord of guilt in her that would compel her to stay – at least long enough for us to talk.

So I closed up the shop and drove from Inglewood to San Gabriel (we had moved there thinking a geographical escape would be the answer to our problems). My mind was racing as the elation of the new life I was contemplating was suddenly being turned into devastation. I hung onto the hope that I would be able to convince her to give me one last chance. As I got off the freeway, my anticipation level was almost unbearable. I really didn't think she would actually leave, but the small chance she would be gone scared the heck out of me. I pulled around the corner where we lived fully expecting to see her car sitting there. But to my astonishment, she was gone. Oh my God! I didn't know what to do. I walked into the house and found a "Dear John" note. Nothing I read gave me any hope that this was simply a temporary situation. At the end of the note were some referrals for treatment centers that might be able to help me if that was something I wanted to pursue. The letter in no way gave me hope that if I got help she would return. I was devastated. I went to the back door to get some love from my two pit bulls and, as the three of us sat down on the couch, I sadly informed them, "Your Mommy's gone," and burst into tears.

After going on a weeklong binge filled with alternating grief and anger, I decided to pursue recovery in an attempt to save my marriage. I called the pastor of my church who told me that the treatment center at Robert F. Kennedy Hospital in Hawthorne, California had a good reputation. I remember how nervous I was when making the call to the hospital, but was grateful when the guy who answered was warm and friendly. I asked about the program and he informed me of the different levels of care they offered. The outpatient program appeared to be the best option, as it would allow me to work.

I made an appointment to be assessed and started that evening. I felt very good about myself and proudly called Robin to let her know I had entered a treatment program and that she could now come home. Much to my disappointment and anger, she stated she would not. Furthermore, she had been instructed by *my* counselors not to talk to me about our relationship until we could do it with a counselor present. Now this really ticked me off! What did they think they were doing meddling in my personal affairs? They had no right! I called the treatment center immediately and asked to speak with the person responsible. A man named Jim got on the phone and calmly tried to explain to me that it was best to do it this way and to give Robin some time. He also stated we could get together to talk on Friday. Although I did not approve of this, it appeared I had no choice. I now held onto Friday as the day my wife would come back to me. I continued in the program motivated by that thought.

When Friday came, I had three full days of sobriety and was very excited about our meeting. I called the center to speak with Jim to verify our appointment and was told that we didn't have one. I blew up! I hung up the phone very angry and confused. I felt betrayed by that counselor (even though today I realize I may have simply heard what I wanted to hear and we really never did firm up a time for the appointment). Anyway, in my anger I left work and went straight to Robin's folks' house where she was staying and begged her to come back to me. I burst into tears attempting to make her feel guilty so she would return home to me. My plea sounded something like this; "I've done what I needed to do by getting into treatment and all you can do is listen to those damn counselors!" I often joke with my friends as I recount those events, "If I were her, I would have felt sorry for me." I also believe I was seeking my mother-in-law's sympathy as she had a tendency to minimize problems in the family and maybe she would get Robin to see things my way. However, Robin remained unscathed and "stuck to her guns." She was going to listen to those counselors, and that was that. I then flew into a rage and told her I wanted a divorce. I then made a violent exit by slamming my in-laws' door, shaking the whole house.

I found myself at one of the biggest crossroads of my life. I was far too upset to return to work, and felt I had only two options: I was going to get seriously loaded, or I was going to the treatment center to reach out for help. It was at this point the miracle in my life began to happen. I actually made a decision to go to the treatment center to talk with somebody, anybody who would listen. To this day, I am still amazed a guy with only three days of sobriety was able to pass up a perfectly justifiable reason to use in favor of reaching out for help – something I was not very good at.

When I arrived at the center, Jack, a patient in the inpatient program, greeted me. He sensed I was in trouble and proceeded to help me calm down. One of the counselors eventually approached and asked me what was happening. I briefed him about my anger towards Jim, the counselor whom I felt had lied to me. I was directed into the group room to wait for Jim who was willing to talk with me. Approximately ten minutes passed and I was getting angry again. I couldn't wait to give him a piece of my mind.

Finally, a very small man who walked as if he were ten feet tall entered the room. It was not that he appeared cocky, but he was very confident as he walked into the room. He had an uncanny look of serenity on his face – especially considering our imminent confrontation. Just as I was getting ready to lay into him, he asked me in a very calm voice, "Are you angry with me?" To this day, I don't know what it was about the way he said those words, but they seemed to handcuff me. All of the energy I had saved up to attack him seemed to have been drained out of me. I guess I wasn't used to that type of honest, straightforward inquiry. All I could say, very meekly, was, "Uh, well yeah." I proceeded to let him know why I was so angry, but it lacked the punch I had originally intended. After he very deliberately told me we had never actually scheduled a session, he asked me to follow him into the other room. I was curious and nervous about where he might be leading me.

We approached a closed door and my curiosity grew. He swung the door open and my heart dropped as I found my outpatient counselor, Kay, and Robin sitting in a very small office. Jim stated, "Okay, you want to talk? Let's talk." At this point, I was feeling completely powerless. I knew there was great power in the room and none of it was mine. I also knew there was nothing I could say that would result in my wife coming home any time soon. They sensed my lack of power and Jim proceeded to let me know, in a very loving manner, that I was no longer appropriate for the outpatient program and they needed me to transition into the inpatient program. It was clear, from the faces of everyone in the room, that getting me to agree to inpatient treatment was the purpose of this meeting.

After the initial shock wore off, I proceeded to tell them all the reasons why this couldn't possibly work – especially because my Dad needed me at work (although at that point I was not nearly the exemplary worker I used to be). They were not fazed by my response and held firm. I still would not agree. There was no way I was "going inpatient." After all, I hadn't even relapsed. It appeared they were ready to give up on trying to change my mind when Jim said to me, "We're going to leave the room now to give you some time alone to think about it. We really hope you decide to stay with us." They all left the room.

There I sat, just me and God (although I wasn't aware of His presence at that time). I no longer had anyone to argue with. My mind raced. I wondered how all my good intentions had blown up in my face. I wondered why I had not given Jim a piece of my mind. I wondered why I could not get my wife turned around on this thing. I wondered what living in an inpatient setting would be like. I wondered how my Dad would be able run the business without me. And, finally, I wondered why I was now considering entering the inpatient program. It was at this moment, sitting alone in that room, when the biggest miracle and turning point in my life happened. I found myself completely surrendered to what other people thought was best for me. I had decided I would enter the inpatient program against my better judgment. Amazing!

My only explanation for the scenario just described is God was working in my life. To this day, I am amazed at the turn of events. I went from thinking I was getting my wife back that day, to being on the edge of relapse. It was also the day Jim, an amazing counselor and interventionist, entered my life. He made all the right moves in setting me up for the miracle that resulted in my doing something I was vehemently against, but desperately needed at that point in my life.

It is obvious a miracle was working in Robin's life as well. She had never before exhibited the strength to resist my manipulation and, over those few days, was able to take suggestions from others to do things that were very difficult for her to do. I was very angry with her at the time, but now see her actions as critical elements in saving my life.

I guess I thought by going into treatment, the counselors would simply hit me with the magic sobriety wand and I would be stricken sober. Little did I know the counselors didn't do it for me at all. What they did was teach *me* how to do it. This is what I hope you'll learn by reading this book.

In over twenty years of working with people addicted to alcohol and drugs, I have seen many people succeed, and fail, in getting sober and staying sober. There are easily identifiable reasons for these successes and failures in recovery. In a nutshell, those who are able to stay sober follow the recipe for recovery, and those who continue to relapse do not.

When I say *recipe*, I am not talking about what the author thinks is a good idea for recovery. I am talking about what most people who have had experience in working with alcoholics and addicts, and those who have had success in recovery, recommend.

Whether they know it or not, most patients who enter a chemical de-pendence treatment center are making the statement, "I don't know what the heck I'm doing when it comes to sobriety, so please show me how to do it." This is the best attitude you can have in reading this book. Leave your ideas at the door. If you knew what you were doing in regard to sobriety you wouldn't need to read it.

The information presented here is mainstream information regarding sobriety. It forms the foundation for countless treatment programs across the country. This information is what you purchase when you spend thousands of dollars entering a treatment center. Don't get me wrong – I very much believe in chemical dependency treatment and it was instrumental in saving my own life. However, not everyone has the resources for such an expense, and many state and county-funded programs are difficult to access. This is my primary purpose for writ-ing this book.

If you are truly ready to stop the madness of your drug and alcohol abuse, then it is time to follow the principles presented here. Remem-ber, the people who get sober are those who follow what has worked for others. Those who don't, continue drinking or using. It's just that simple! People don't come up to me after a relapse and say, "Bob, I did x, y, and z and I still got loaded!" What they tell me is something like, "Well, I was doing x and y, but wasn't doing z" or, "I was doing x, y, and z, but stopped doing x." Thus, they weren't following the recipe for recovery and/or they got complacent.

The fact you are reading this book indicates, at least on some level, your desire for a new life. For that, I want to congratulate you. Some people never make it this far. Now the real work starts. For people to be successful in recovery, they need to want it so badly that they are willing to go to any lengths to get it. I hope you are at that place. What that attitude will translate into is the willingness to follow these suggestions. No matter what you think (and remember you're thinking at this point with an addicted mind), **none of the suggestions in this book are outlandish!** This stuff is mainstream sobriety and it is what most people do who have success in recovery. Now you must decide whom to listen to – what you think, or what successful people in sobriety think. As some in the program say, "Your best thinking got you here." I sincerely hope you're ready to follow the directions this book provides and get your life back.

The book initially focuses on the *problem* of alcoholism/addiction. This will help you learn about the disease model of alcoholism/addiction and to determine whether or not you're an addict/alcoholic. This is followed by a chapter entitled "The Solution" which contains concrete ingredients for recovery – the things to *do* if you want to stay sober. At the end of that chapter, you will find a simple-to-use Sobriety Checklist. Use this tool to help you track your progress while reading the next chapter, "Getting Started," which will help you do just that. Then you will find a chapter with still more ingredients for recovery. Next, we will visit relapse prevention where you will learn how to better anticipate relapse and how to stop it. This is followed by a tour through the 12 Steps of Alcoholics Anonymous – a path to recovery that is also used by other 12-Step programs like Narcotics Anonymous, Marijuana Anonymous, Cocaine Anonymous, and Crystal Meth Anonymous. We will then focus on how to deal with uncomfortable feelings that alcoholics and drug addicts escape from by using their substance of choice. We conclude with a chapter that will help you structure recovery into your daily living and a chapter that reveals some of the miracles I have seen and experienced in recovery. Now, let's get started with your new life.

Please note: As you will see in the first chapter, alcoholism and drug addiction are the same problem. Alcohol *is* a drug and, if you are an alcoholic, you are "addicted" to alcohol. Consequently, and for ease of writing, I will be using the terms alcoholic and drug addict, and alcoholism and addiction, interchangeably. Simply apply the solution to your substance of choice. You will also find that there is a spiritual (not religious) component to recovery in which I will use the terms God and Higher Power interchangeably – not to impose my personal beliefs, but simply for ease of writing. Finally, you will notice that many paragraphs in the book are italicized. I have also done this for ease of reading as I switch from teaching recovery principles (normal type) to demonstrating how many of these principles were effective in saving my own life and the lives of others (*italics*).

CHAPTER 1
THE PROBLEM

Before getting into the solution, the primary focus of this book, it is important to understand what we are dealing with. I will avoid going into great depth here because I don't want you to get bogged down with the vast quantities of information available on this subject. After all, the reason you picked up this book is that you have likely come to the conclusion that alcohol and/or drugs are having an adverse affect on you and those around you. Understanding the cause of your situation is helpful, but it is the solution that will ultimately make you well. I will outline on these pages what I, and thousands like me in my profession, think is important for you to know at this point regarding the *disease* of alcoholism/addiction.

People who do not suffer from addiction cannot possibly understand why we continue to use when it results in such a mess. They might ask themselves, "Why don't these people just pull up their bootstraps and get their act together?" Since our addiction often leads us to immoral behavior and continued use despite the pain we cause ourselves and others, we are often seen as bad, immoral people. Therefore, when we try to stop, we are often viewed as bad people trying to get good. Fed this message by society, and perhaps believing it ourselves, we reach for our bootstraps and, inevitably, fail miserably. It is virtually impossible to take this "moral" view of addiction and recover. Again, I know this from personal experience and from over two decades of helping recovering addicts fight their addiction. With this information, it becomes obvious you must take a different view of the problem if you are to recover.

The Disease Model

Despite what you and others may believe about this problem, I have something very important to tell you: you are not a bad person trying to get good – *you are a sick person trying to get well.* This *disease model* is the predominate view of those who treat this problem. E. M. Jelinek, considered "the father of alcohol studies in the United States," aided the shift from the moral model to the disease model of addiction (Kinney and

> You are not a bad person trying to get good – you are a sick person trying to get well.

Leaton, 1987, pp. 52-53). He essentially came to the conclusion that, "Hey, world, you mislabeled this thing. You put it in the sin bin, and it really belongs on the disease pile" (Kinney and Leaton, 1987, p. 53). Terence Gorski, a pioneer in the field of relapse prevention, wrote a book with Merlene Miller called *Staying Sober*, a book I highly recommend. In this book, he lists the many professional organizations that accept the disease model of alcoholism:

> The work of E. M. Jelinek in the '50s and '60s led to acceptance of alcoholism as a disease by the American Medical Association, the American Medical Society on Alcoholism, the National Counsel on Alcoholism, the American Psychiatric Association, and the American Academy of Family Practice. It is also considered a disease by the American Psychological Association, American Public Health Association, American Hospital Association, and the World Health Organization (Gorski and Miller, 1986, p. 40).

Despite what I previously thought about this problem, these organizations have likely invested much time and research in reaching this controversial conclusion. It was much more beneficial for me to take their word for it than to assume I knew better than they.

Dr. William Silkworth wrote a letter for use in the book, *Alcoholics Anonymous,* commonly known as the "Big Book," in which he describes alcoholism as an allergy:

...the action of alcohol on these chronic alcoholics is a manifestation of an allergy; the phenomenon of craving is limited to this class and never occurs in the average temperate drinker. These allergic types can never safely use alcohol in any form at all... . Frothy emotional appeal seldom suffices... After they have succumbed to the desire again, as so many do, and the phenomenon of craving develops, they pass through the well-known stages of a spree, emerging remorseful, with a firm resolution not to drink again. This is repeated over and over, and unless this person can experience an entire psychic change, there is very little hope for his recovery.

On the other hand – and strange as it may seem to those who do not understand – once a psychic change has occurred, the very same person who seemed doomed... suddenly finds himself easily able to control his desire for alcohol, the only effort necessary being that required to follow a few certain rules (Alcoholics Anonymous, 2001, p. xxviii-xxix).

The rules he is speaking of apply to all addictions and are found in the program of recovery as outlined in *Alcoholics Anonymous*. Remember, we are using the term alcoholism here, but the principles we are discussing also apply to other drugs.

This disease model of alcoholism has many positive implications for those who suffer from it. First, we no longer have to be so hard on ourselves for having it. Alcoholism and addiction are diseases, which puts them in the same class as diabetes and cancer. Asking an alcoholic to just stop drinking is like asking a cancer patient to just control its spread.

Next, the disease model allows us to begin breaking the addiction cycle (see Figure 1 on the next page). The cycle starts with an uncomfortable feeling. Alcoholics and addicts don't do well with feelings and have the need to escape from them. This leads to craving the chemical of choice – the source of relief from emotional pain. The craving, in turn, leads to eventual use of the drug. For the alcoholic/addict, this use inevitably leads to negative consequences. As a result, uncomfortable feelings (often shame and guilt) return and, thus, the cycle begins again. The primary way of breaking the addiction cycle is for alcoholics/addicts to develop recovery tools that will allow them to work through the uncomfortable feelings. We will discuss this later in the book. Another way to interrupt the cycle is to decrease the shame and guilt associated with using. The disease model allows for this. When addicts understand they are sick people trying to get well rather than bad people trying to get good, the shame associated with being an addict significantly decreases. Thus, by decreasing the shame and guilt associated with using, the cycle is disrupted.

Figure 1

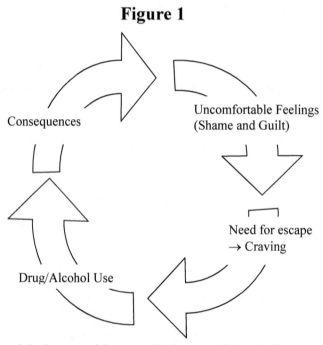

The disease model also provides us with hope. If alcoholism is a moral issue, as many have viewed it in the past, then we feel that becoming better people should solve the problem. So we set out to be upstanding citizens by just stopping our immoral behavior. We have repeatedly proven to ourselves and others that this solution has no chance of working. Therefore, we fail at becoming moral people, believe we are bad, and feel there is no hope. The disease model implies we need outside help just as we would with other diseases like diabetes or cancer. This perceived need for outside help not only provides us with renewed hope, but is also the key to entering and maintaining our recovery.

> This is an "I can't" but "we can" addiction.

This is an "I can't" but "we can" addiction (Gorski, 1989). When we begin getting into the solution in the next chapter, you will see this "we can" solution as the over-riding theme of everything we do to get and stay sober.

Where Does This Disease Come From?

There has been much discussion about what causes the disease of addiction. Many believe genetics are involved. It is a well-known fact that those who have parents, grandparents and/or other family members who are alcoholics have a much higher chance of developing alcoholism than those who do not. Others believe the disease arises from psychological factors such as the impact of parental upbringing on self-esteem and the person's inability to manage uncomfortable emotions. Still others believe it arises from social causes – social influences that contribute to the development of the disease. I believe all of the above are true and subscribe to the biopsychosocial model of addiction. I strongly believe all of these factors contribute to its development and are intertwined. I also believe there is a very strong spiritual component – lacking an awareness of the existence of greater meaning in life than what is readily apparent.

Understanding and accepting addiction as a disease may be a novel idea to you and may perhaps be a little difficult to accept. However, millions of recovering alcoholics and addicts have bought into this idea and have found a solution. Your old views have not worked for you and subscribing to this view has worked for many. So begin to get rid of some of your old ideas and replace them with new ideas that have a chance to save your life! At this point I want to share with you some other views I have about the disease of addiction that are widely accepted by many others who work in this profession, and by those who have recovered.

I firmly believe alcoholics and drug addicts are highly sensitive people. Things tend to bother us more than most people and we worry about whatever is bothering us to the point we become obsessed by it. Compounding this problem, we are also inherently intolerant of emotion. When a feeling arises, our first impulse is to suppress it. So, not only do we worry more in quantity and intensity, we are not equipped like others to deal with such emotion. Therefore, when we stumble upon drugs and alcohol, and find they enable us to avoid feelings, our reaction is typically "Eureka!" From then on, we know an escape from our feelings is as easy as using drugs or alcohol. It happens just that quickly for many of us.

I also believe addiction develops for some of us at a much slower pace. Such people might engage in the social norm of going out on Saturday nights and having a couple drinks. It is done very innocently and consequences may not surface. However, I believe a message is implanted into the subconscious that reads, "Hmm, when I have those couple of drinks on Saturday nights, I feel really with it – ready to have the time of my life." They might decide since it worked on Saturday night, why not Friday night too? Again, the subconscious mind gets the message, "Hmm, when I have alcohol on those evenings, I feel no pain." Then they might have a difficult day at work and it suddenly occurs to them that a drink sounds good. They don't consciously know they are killing emotional pain at this point and they decide to have that drink. Again, the subconscious gets a similar message. Then they might have a bad day and say to themselves, "I need a drink." At this point, the subconscious belief that drinking and using makes life better has moved to conscious awareness and they now know exactly what they are doing – gaining relief from a lousy feeling. The disease progresses as the person runs to drugs and/or alcohol whenever an uncomfortable feeling develops. Since the person realizes these substances work quickly and efficiently, any healthy ways of dealing with uncomfortable feelings that may have been used in the past are quickly forgotten. Soon, the only option the person has to gain relief is to drink or use.

Do You Have the Disease of Addiction?

Now that we have explored the disease model of addiction, you might still be wondering if you, in fact, have the disease. An important indicator of addiction is whether or not you continue to drink or use despite negative consequences. These consequences can involve the following:

- Marital or relationship problems
- Work problems
- Health problems
- Legal problems
- Dishonesty
- Emotional turmoil
- Emotional absence or neglect of children
- Giving up hobbies or recreational activities
- Financial difficulties
- Acting against your personal morals
- Social isolation
- Poor hygiene
- Becoming irresponsible
- Breaking promises
- Quick temper

Non-addicted people will look at all these bad things happening, realize they are hurting themselves or others, and simply stop using. Addicts and alcoholics will look at such consequences, make a decision to stop using, and eventually return to use despite the consequences.

Failed attempts at stopping use are also strong indicators of addiction. Most addicts who eventually seek outside help have had repeated attempts at quitting. Often they have some success at remaining off their drug of choice for extended periods of time. Such apparent success is often mistaken for non-addiction. They say to themselves, "See, I have proven that I am not an addict because I have remained off drugs for 'x' amount of time." Having mistakenly proven their non-addiction to themselves, they return to use and create more consequences. Others have very little success at quitting for any significant period of time. Such people may actually be better off because they recognize the need for help sooner and get busy seeking ways to recover.

Another strong indicator of addiction is using more than you intended. Almost every time I used drugs or alcohol, I intended to use an amount that would result in minimal consequences. I failed almost every time at sticking to such a plan. Despite having proven repeatedly that I could not limit my use, I was surprised every time I failed. My failure was most likely due to the phenomenon of craving described by Dr. Silkworth that was mentioned earlier. Once I began using, the phenomenon of craving kicked in and I was utterly powerless over continued use. Therefore, I firmly believe complete abstinence can be the only successful way to be relieved of addiction. As noted above, Dr. Silkworth concurs.

> ...I firmly believe that complete abstinence can be the only successful way to be relieved of addiction.

I have seen many people unsuccessfully attempt to cut down or to learn controlled drinking. However, some researchers have actually claimed success at teaching clients how to do so. Kinney and Leaton (1987) cite a famous study by Linda and Mark Sobell in which it appeared they were successfully teaching alcoholics controlled drinking. "The initial reports were quite positive, they claimed" (p. 271). However, "Several researchers very painstakingly tracked down the subjects of the Sobells' study to see how they had fared over the long haul. Of the original group, only one was described as continuing as a moderate drinker. All of the others had serious problems and relapses, and four had died of alcohol-related problems" (p. 272).

A few years ago, I was watching a television show (20/20) in which the host was interviewing a woman who was the founder of a controlled drinking program. She claimed they were successfully teaching clients controlled drinking. As I listened to this woman, I could feel the hair on the back of my head stand up because there were probably many alcoholics watching the show who were buying into this. Due to what I know about the disease, it deeply saddened and angered me that some alcoholics might have their recovery postponed because of this bad information. What I know about this disease was re-confirmed only weeks later.

In July of 2000, I attended the International Convention of Alcoholics Anonymous in Minneapolis with my brother, Ken, who also has significant sober time in the program. It was a wonderful experience as we joined approximately 50,000 other alcoholics in Minneapolis, Minnesota, celebrating recovery. We virtually filled the Metrodome at the

Friday night meeting and spirituality was in the air. We were both very touched by this celebration and wished it could have lasted longer.

As we waited for our return flight at the airport in Minneapolis, a friend we met at the convention handed me a newspaper article featuring the same woman from the television show who had promoted controlled drinking. Unfortunately, the article indicated that this woman had been arrested for manslaughter after she killed an entire family while driving drunk! So much for controlled drinking. I can't help but feel sad for this woman I had resented just weeks earlier, and for the victims of her drinking episode. Her consequences are so severe that she will probably be in jail too long to ever know the gifts of true recovery. But the gifts of recovery can belong to you if you act before it is too late.

What Kind of an Alcoholic or Addict are You?

To continue our discussion of whether or not you are an alcoholic and/or addict, it is important for you to know there are many different types of alcoholics and addicts. Are you the type who drinks or uses all day, every day, and/or must do so to avoid withdrawal symptoms and stay well? To most, this is the stereotypical alcoholic. Some such alcoholics end up unemployed and homeless. However, some alcoholics of this type are able to keep their jobs and family. They often fool themselves into believing they are not alcoholics because they compare themselves to "gutter drunks." But they are very much alcoholics because alcohol has control over their lives.

Are you an alcoholic/addict who is in denial because you only drink at night after work to unwind? You appear to have the ability to abstain during the day, but are compelled to drink every night. Not every person who does this is alcoholic, but if you have some of the consequences mentioned previously and you do not, or cannot, stop this pattern, you are certainly an alcoholic. You might also compare yourself to the gutter drunk, which keeps you sick until you face the truth about your condition.

Are you a person who uses only on weekends, but you use enough to result in negative consequences? Despite such consequences, the disease will also have you believe that you are not alcoholic because you don't drink every day or because you are able to hang onto your family or job.

Finally, are you a "periodic" or "binge" drinker who can go weeks, or even months without drinking? You have periodic sprees in which you binge for days or weeks and have many consequences. It is particularly difficult for you to come to terms with your addiction because, every time you stop using after a binge, you view such temporary success as evidence of non-addiction – especially if you compare yourself to the gutter drunk.

I hope this discussion on the types of addiction prevents you from being fooled about your drinking or using. No matter what your pattern, if you continue to drink or use despite negative consequences, you are most assuredly addicted. If you continue to have questions about whether or not you are an alcoholic/addict, I invite you to take a standardized test called the CAGE, which might aid you in coming to the appropriate conclusion. According to Kinney and Leaton (1987):

> No matter what your pattern, if you continue to drink despite negative consequences, you are most assuredly addicted.

> Since its introduction in 1970, the CAGE developed by Ewing and Rouse has become recognized as one of the most efficient and effective screening devices. It consists of four questions which are as follows:
>
> - Have you ever felt you should *Cut* down on your drinking?
> - Have people *Annoyed* you by criticizing your drinking?
> - Have you ever felt bad or *Guilty* about your drinking?
> - Have you ever had a drink first thing in the morning to steady nerves or get rid of a hangover? (*Eye*-opener)

Two or three affirmative answers should create a high index of suspicion. Four positive responses indicate alcoholism (p. 184).

Although this questionnaire was developed as a screening tool for alcoholism, multiple positive answers for a drug user should also provide a high suspicion of problem use. If you are an alcoholic or a drug addict, it is very important you eventually come to this conclusion yourself. We who work in the addiction profession often refer to it as the only self-diagnosed disease. I can tell you that you are an alcoholic "until the cows come home", but unless you believe it, you will not seek help.

As we now turn to the solution in the next chapter, it is important for you to know that most people who enter into recovery from alcoholism and addiction do relapse. I tell you this not to discourage you, but to let you know that recovery takes a lot of work and persistence. As it states in *Alcoholics Anonymous*, the basic text of Alcoholics Anonymous: "Half measures availed us nothing" (*Alcoholics Anonymous*, 2001, p. 59). You must give yourself completely to recovery if you are to succeed. Those who relapse are typically those who continue to try to do it their way or start to get well too soon and stop doing the things that got them sober. Those who achieve long-term sobriety without relapse are those who follow the recipe and stay persistent. At the risk of giving you permission to relapse, it is also important for you to know that relapse is not necessarily a sign that the program is not working for you. It is, however, a wake-up call that you may not be doing all you need to do to abstain from drugs or alcohol. Recovery is a process, not a destination.

> Recovery is a process, not a destination.

As you move along in recovery, you will progressively become more comfortable with yourself and your recovery. The road to recovery is wondrous and I invite you to trust the process of recovery you are about to learn. It will work for you if you want it to and sometimes if you're not sure you want it. So hang on to your seat – you're in for a great ride.

CHAPTER 2
THE SOLUTION:
INGREDIENTS FOR RECOVERY

What will become obvious very quickly as you read the following recipe for recovery is that it takes quite a commitment to get and stay sober. In fact, sobriety will have to be considered by you the number one priority in your life in order for you to be willing to follow these suggestions. Many of us have ruined our lives to the point that we are willing to take any suggestion if we can just regain control. Others who have not had such severe consequences yet ("yet" being the key word here) may find it more difficult to make sobriety their number one priority. I hope you can learn from those who have gone before you on the path of recovery. The lesson here is that your chances for recovery will be greatly diminished if sobriety is not the most important thing in your life. If you really think about it, without sobriety you will eventually lose those things on which you may be placing a higher priority, such as job, money, health, hobbies, or family. Simply put, if you have sobriety you will likely be able to hold onto those things you cherish. Without sobriety, you will surely lose them.

With this in mind, let us look at the ingredients for recovery which will most surely change your life. As each new ingredient for recovery is listed below, it will be highlighted. These highlighted ingredients and others can be found on a single list at the end of the chapter. I encourage you to make a copy of this list for your quick reference as you work your program of recovery so you can gauge how you're doing. In this chapter, we will focus on the ingredients related to working a strong 12-Step program. In Chapter 4, you'll read about some additional ingredients for recovery.

Detox Warning: If you have decided to get sober and are planning on discontinuing your use of alcohol and/or other drugs, please read the brief section on detoxification near the beginning of Chapter 3 to learn about whom you can consult to determine if you need a medically supervised detox. It is important to note that discontinuing certain drugs including, but not limited to, alcohol, benzodiazapines, barbiturates, GHB, and some of the newer designer drugs can be fatal if not under the care of a physician. Be sure to contact a physician or an alcohol and drug treatment center if you have any questions regarding the level of risk involved in discontinuing your drug of choice.

12-Step Meetings

Alcoholics Anonymous (AA), Narcotics Anonymous (NA), Cocaine Anonymous (CA), Marijuana Anonymous (MA), Crystal Meth Anonymous (CMA), and similar organizations are all examples of 12-Step programs. Such programs use the 12 Steps, which were originally written for the AA program. These steps have been the key to a life without drugs and alcohol for millions of people around the world. We will cover the 12 Steps in Chapter 6.

For now, you need to get started with **meeting attendance** as soon as possible. At these meetings you will hear what others have done to achieve successful recovery. It is also at these meetings that you will begin to develop your sober support system. Meetings can be found by simply calling the central office of the program of your choice and asking where and when the local meetings are held. The local telephone numbers for AA and NA can typically be found in the phone book. If you want to contact one of the other anonymous programs, the AA or NA office will usually be able to direct you to them. You can also get the numbers by calling your local alcohol and drug treatment center – also found in the phone book. I have included the phone numbers and websites of the national offices of many of the 12 Step programs, along with other resources in Appendix 2 near the end of the book. Meetings can be found in most cities at multiple times during the day and evening hours. When you go to a meeting, pick up a meeting directory so you can plan which meetings you will go to next.

The most common suggestion regarding the number of meetings a newcomer should attend is 90 meetings in your first 90 days. This was suggested to me in my early recovery and I complied because, by the time I got to the program, I was truly ready to follow direction from those who knew more than I about sobriety. Some of the reasoning behind this suggestion is that in the first three months of daily meeting attendance you will learn what you need to know to stay sober. Another reason that was presented to me is it takes ten to twelve weeks to develop new habits. Developing the habit of addressing my recovery on a daily basis was very important for me as I have a tendency to become easily distracted.

If you have just recently made a decision to begin a program of recovery, such a commitment might seem overwhelming to you. It was helpful for me to apply the commonly used phrase in AA, "One Day at a Time." Using this principle, instead of "90 in 90," it becomes just a meeting today. So all you have to do to keep this commitment is to go to a meeting today. Worry about tomorrow's meeting tomorrow. Also, if you have bought into the necessity of making sobriety your number one priority, an hour and a half out of your day for something so important should not be asking too much of yourself.

Another very important reason for daily meetings in early recovery is it is much easier to adjust down the number of meetings you are attending than to adjust up:

When I completed my 90 in 90, I went to my sponsor (a mentor or guide in recovery) and asked "What now?" He asked me if I was sure I was ready to cut down on my meetings; after all, things were going well and I had not relapsed. I felt he made a good point and decided not to make a change yet. After another month, I decided it was time to cut down and my sponsor agreed. He suggested I try six meetings weekly for a while to see how I felt. I did this for three weeks and my sponsor and I agreed that I could drop down to five weekly. When I eventually dropped down to four meetings per week, it did not feel quite right so I stepped it back up to five weekly and again felt comfortable. It was easy for me to step back up to five since I had created room in my life for daily meetings previously. Had I only started off going to three meetings weekly and decided my comfort zone was not adequate, it would have been much more difficult for me to adjust my schedule enough to increase my attendance. Daily meetings also allowed me to begin my sobriety at a higher comfort level so I knew what kind of serenity was available to me.

Finally, I make this suggestion based not only on the experience of my personal recovery, but on my professional experience as well. When patients enter our treatment center, one of the most important goals I have is to get them to see the importance of daily meetings and to convince them to do 90 in 90. This is due to the fact I have seen that, those who do so, have higher rates of success than those who don't. As mentioned above, most people who enter recovery eventually relapse. I realize this is a very scary thought, but the chances for long-term, relapse-free recovery is much higher for those who follow the recipe you are reading now. Again, my intent in bringing this up is to motivate you enough to be in the group that gets it the first time. It is truly in your grasp if you are willing to take direction.

The next suggestion regarding meeting attendance is to attend the same meetings every week – for example, you have a regular Monday meeting, Tuesday meeting, etc. If you don't particularly care for a given meeting, find another and go to that one every week. By having such consistency at meetings, you will begin developing acquaintances, and even friendships, at the meetings. Since one of the difficulties for newcomers is that they are going to a meeting full of strangers, knowing people there makes it easier to attend.

There are many different formats that 12-Step meetings follow and I recommend attending at least 50% "sharing" or "discussion" meetings. In such meetings, people open up about their struggles and successes in recovery. At speaker meetings, a person with significant sober time shares what it was like drinking or using, what happened that prompted recovery, and what life is like being sober. Although such meetings are very valuable, if you attend only those meetings, it is too easy to hide and go unnoticed. You should also attend at least one Big Book Study or Step Study meeting. In a Big Book Study, a specific portion of the Big Book (*Alcoholics Anonymous, Narcotics Anonymous,* etc.) is read and discussed. In a Step Study, one of the 12 Steps is read and discussed from *12 Steps and 12 Traditions* (1987), commonly known as the "12 and 12." This is a good way to get a better understanding of how to work the steps and the benefits of doing so.

Lastly, you should attend at least one gender specific meeting in which only members of the same sex attend. I find these to be the best meetings due to the lack of distraction of the opposite sex and the high level of honesty that is particularly evident in such meetings. When you obtain a meeting directory, it is very simple to identify different meeting formats because of the code next to each meeting listing, i.e. SS = Step Study, W = Women Only, and S = Speaker Meeting.

As mentioned near the start of this chapter, there are many different types of 12-Step meetings. Alcoholics Anonymous, NA, CA, MA, CMA, and PA (Pills Anonymous) are all 12-Step programs. The school of thought is you should attend the meeting that matches your drug of choice. I take a rather controversial stance regarding this issue. It is based on the fact that, whether you are addicted to alcohol, narcotics, cocaine, marijuana, or pills, addiction is addiction. So it should not matter which recovery meeting you go to. Different people will feel comfortable in different meetings.

Although cocaine was the drug that caused me the most trouble, I felt most comfortable in AA. I felt I fit into those meetings more than I did in CA. This may have been due to the fact that in the particular CA meetings I attended, people shared about their experience with cocaine more graphically than I was comfortable with. When cocaine was talked about in that way, it triggered me to want to use. Additionally, in the meetings I was exposed to, there appeared to be more sobriety in AA than CA, and less relapse. This is not to say that this is true across the board, but it was true at the meetings I was exposed to. I have since discovered that there are CA meetings in which there is significant sobriety and you may be fortunate enough to find them in your early recovery if you are addicted to cocaine. The bottom line here is that I recommend attending the meetings that you feel will give you the best chance at sobriety.

In my estimation, the key to identifying a good meeting is by measuring the degree to which the solution is talked about instead of the problem. We all know what the problem is. It is important the problem is talked about to some degree so people, especially newcomers, can identify with others' problems. But such discussion should be followed by a discussion of what the person is doing, or has done, about the problem. Nothing bothers me more than attending a meeting where people share every week about the same problem in recovery, but do not share what they are doing about it.

Another strong indicator of a good meeting is if members put their hand out to newcomers. At the start of meetings, newcomers are asked to identify themselves. This enables other members of the group to know who the newcomers are. If you go to a meeting and identify yourself as a newcomer, other members will introduce themselves and welcome you to the meeting. If they don't, you might want to find another meeting.

Sharing at meetings is another very important suggestion because it is a good way for people to get to know you so you can build a sober support system. Don't worry if you feel you don't have anything to share. A very acceptable share is as follows: "Hi. My name is Bob and I'm an alcoholic. I have five days of sobriety. I don't really have anything to share, but someone suggested that I share at meetings so that's what I'm doing. That's all I have to share." You will be amazed at the results of such a simple share. People will introduce themselves to you after the meeting and likely provide support and maybe even their phone number. Again, if nobody does this, it is a sign that you are probably not at a very good meeting and you might want to find another.

Meeting commitments are recommended as well in early recovery. People take commitments for such things as set-up, clean up, coffee person, treasurer, literature person, secretary, and greeter, among others. The benefit of taking a commitment is that, if there is a time that you're feeling lazy or unmotivated to go to a meeting, you go anyway because others are counting on you to be there to fulfill your commitment. In my experience, even if I go for that reason alone, I am always happy I attended. It is also a good way to get other people to know you because those with commitments are recognized for their efforts toward the end of the meeting. It also makes you feel connected to the meeting and to AA as a whole. Most successful members of AA will also tell you that **being of service** inherently helps you stay sober. I agree.

It is important to be **punctual at meetings,** so try to be on time and don't leave early. It is actually a good idea to be early, and stay for a while after the meeting, as this furthers your opportunities to meet people and to build your sober support system. Many meetings offer **fellowship** afterward in which members meet at a regular spot, usually a restaurant, for food or coffee. This is still another way to build your sober support system.

Developing a 12-Step sober support system of peers is very important in recovery and attending the same meetings every week will enable you to do that. One of the essential components of my early sobriety was meeting and hanging out with people in the program with whom I could relate. I met a group of guys that I had a lot in common with. We were close to the same age, had similar experiences, and had a good (perhaps sick) sense of humor. The "AA Team," as they called themselves, welcomed me with open arms. We went to meetings, shared our stories with program newcomers at the rehab center (aka 12-Step panels), and hung out with each other before and after such functions. I am extremely grateful for those guys as they made me feel part of the group and kept me busy in my early sobriety. I have made many sober friends since, and I still have a home group to which I travel 40 miles each week. There are meetings that are much closer, but the guys at the Redondo Beach Tuesday Men's Stag have a brand of sobriety that is very attractive to me. It is a pleasure to travel that far each week to be with them.

Let us now turn to **sponsorship.** A sponsor is a mentor or guide who will help you along in your sobriety. A sponsor makes suggestions regarding how to work a good program based on his or her own experience. He or she will also provide support during difficult times in sobriety, take you through the basic text of your 12-Step program of choice, and help to guide you through the 12 Steps.

A very common fear that you might have regarding sponsorship is not wanting to burden someone else with your problems. You might feel uncomfortable with the idea of having another person take the time to help you. It is important to know that one alcoholic helping another is the way AA was actually founded: An old friend who was involved with a Christian organization called the Oxford Group visited Bill W., an alcoholic New York stockbroker. As a result of such visits, Bill had what he called a spiritual experience and was staying sober. It was difficult, however, and he wondered how he would keep his sobriety. "He suddenly realized that in order to save himself he must carry his message to another alcoholic" (*Alcoholics Anonymous*, 2001, pp. xv-xvi). He was standing in a hotel lobby and, instead of going into the bar in the next room, called a number from the church directory. "His call to the clergyman led him presently to a certain resident of the town, who, though formerly able and respected, was then nearing the nadir of alcoholic despair" (*Alcoholics Anonymous*, 2001, pp. 154-155). He then paid a visit to this man, Dr. Bob, an Akron physician. This initial meeting between the two men is affectionately known as the first meeting of Alcoholics Anonymous. Dr. Bob became sober, and Bill W. had bought a few more days of sobriety. While the two of them pondered how they might keep their sobriety, they stumbled across another alcoholic whom they helped get sober. As the number of sober alcoholics grew, they realized that helping other alcoholics was what was keeping them sober – and AA was born (*Alcoholics Anonymous*, 2001, pp. xvi-xvii).

Therefore, you should not view sponsorship as a burden but, rather, an essential component of recovery. So instead of burdening the person you are asking to be your sponsor, you are actually aiding him/her to participate in his/her *own* recovery.

I have also found this to be true from personal experience. Before I got into this profession, I worked at my father's print shop and there were days when the stress of the job had my mind far from recovery and in places it shouldn't be. I would suddenly get a call from someone I was sponsoring and it instantly brought my thinking and attitude back into recovery. I would resume working with a renewed attitude of gratitude and serenity.

In selecting a sponsor, you are looking for a person whose sobriety you are attracted to. You might meet a person at a meeting or hear someone share in a way that indicates to you that he or she looks to be in a good mental, emotional and/or spiritual place. If you decide that this brand of sobriety looks attractive to you, and you would like to feel that way in your own recovery, you would ask that person to be your sponsor. Your sponsor will, typically, have you work a sobriety program and work the Steps similar to the way he or she did. It follows that if you work a similar program, and follow your sponsor's direction, you will end up somewhere in the vicinity of the mental, emotional, and spiritual place that attracted you to that person in the first place.

I recommend getting a sponsor within your first 30 days of recovery. If you are having difficulty deciding on a long-term sponsor, you might consider asking someone to be a temporary sponsor. Although it is ideal to have the same sponsor for a long time, you can always change sponsors later if you decide the relationship is not working out.

It is important to select a sponsor of the same sex because nobody can understand a male alcoholic like another male alcoholic. It is the same for women. You should also select someone who has at least a few years of sobriety and who has worked all 12 Steps. As the Big Book states: "…you cannot transmit something you haven't got" (Alcoholics Anonymous, 2001, p. 164). Finally, the person you want as a sponsor should have his or her own sponsor. This is an indication that the person continues to work a strong program of recovery.

It is often difficult to pick up the phone to reach out for help if you're not used to it. For this reason, daily phone calls to your sponsor for the first 90 days are also strongly suggested. If you can force yourself to make a daily call to your sponsor for this period of time, you can break yourself of such hesitancy. As a result, when you really need to call your sponsor for help, you will be able to. Remember, recovery begins with one alcoholic talking to another. Every time you call your sponsor, you are actually helping him or her to stay sober.

Phone calls to your sponsor and other members of your sober support system are vitally important because, as I pointed out earlier, you have proven that you cannot stay sober on your own. You must have others involved in your sobriety if you are to succeed. The more phone calls you make, the better your chances are at continued sobriety (see Appendix 1 near the end

> You must have others involved in your sobriety if you are to succeed.

of the book to find an excellent texting tool). You especially need to call someone when you are feeling as if you want to use, or are feeling particularly stressed or bothered about something. Phone calls that aid in sobriety must be made to other recovering people. Non-recovering people cannot fully understand what you go through as a recovering addict. They don't understand why you don't just get with it and stop using. They also cannot understand your level of sensitivity and lack of ability to tolerate normal human emotion. People in recovery not only understand it, but they are living it and can provide valuable feedback on how to get through the difficult times.

Reading 12-Step literature is another essential tool for recovery. Along with learning how to utilize 12 Step programs to help you get sober, such reading also keeps you in a recovery state of mind and steers you toward new recovery behavior. The most important book for you to read is *Alcoholics Anonymous*, commonly referred to as the "Big Book," and viewed as the "AA Bible" by many. In the first 164 pages, you will find the entire AA program. Bill W. wrote it in 1939 and, in my opinion, was divinely inspired. It is simply amazing to me how insightful this AA co-founder was. The information in that book is just as applicable today as it was then. It is not only to be read, but also to be studied and lived. In fact, many in other anonymous programs read it and apply it to whatever addiction they are battling. I currently attend a weekly Big Book study group in which we read the book for 20 minutes and spend the rest of the meeting discussing what we read. We probably go through the first 164 pages two to three times annually and every time I read the same words, I get something new from them.

The book includes the history of AA, discussion on the disease and symptoms of alcoholism, information about and guidance through the 12 Steps, and information for families and employers of alcoholics. Following the first 164 pages are personal stories of alcoholics, which include: What it was like in their disease, what happened that caused them to get sober, and what their lives are like now. This amazing book can be found at most AA meetings or by calling the AA central office in your area.

Another valued book in the fellowship is *Twelve Steps and Twelve Traditions* (1981), commonly known as the "12 and 12." In this book, the 12 Steps are broken down to give a better understanding of how they work and how to work them. Also included are the all-important 12 Traditions, which have enabled the program to survive since 1935.

Many recovering alcoholics start their day by reading a morning meditation book like *24 Hours a Day, A Day at a Time,* or *Daily Reflections.* For each day of the year, these books provide a brief passage about a given aspect of recovery, a meditation topic, and a prayer. This is a great way to start your day on a spiritual and positive note. It reminds you that your most important task for that particular day is to stay sober.

Working the 12 Steps will result in the peace and serenity necessary for long-term recovery. It will allow you to become comfortable in your own skin. The 12 Steps are a systematic way of developing a spiritual program and a manner of living that holds up to any problem you may be confronted with. The "promises" in the Big Book found on pages 83 and 84 will be fulfilled *only* through working these steps. Specific instructions about how to work the steps can be found in the Big Book, but they have been done in various ways. I recommend following your sponsor's direction in working them so you can attain the same gifts that attracted you to your sponsor.

On the next page is a complete list of the ingredients for recovery. Don't forget to make a copy of the list so you can review it daily. We will review many of the remaining ingredients from this list in Chapter 4.

Ingredients for Recovery

Attend 12-Step meetings

Get a sponsor

Call sponsor

Practice meeting punctuality

Share at meetings

Go to fellowship after meetings

Develop sober support system

Make phone calls

Read 12-Step literature

Get meeting commitments

Work the Steps

Develop spiritual program

Pray

Meditate

Be of service

Avoid drinking/using people

Avoid drinking/using places

Be humble

Journal

Think positive

"Stick with the winners"

Take direction

Don't drink or use

Make sobriety the top priority

Live in the present

Look for similarities

Accept feedback from peers

Write gratitude list

Ask for help

Avoid "stinkin' thinkin'"

Be Honest

Be Open

Be Willing

Get/stay desperate for recovery

Create sobriety plan

Safely dispose of alcohol and drugs

Address other addictive behaviors

Exercise

Get adequate sleep

Use good hygiene

Change bad habits

Eat proper diet

Structure nutrition plan

↓ Caffeine, sugar and fat intake

Develop/resume hobbies

Structure life: work/school/volunteer

Have fun

Avoid unnecessary major changes

Avoid early recovery relationships

Safely dispose of paraphernalia

"Think it through"

Avoid triggers

Be aware of warning signs

Get professional counseling

Consider sober living home

Avoid isolation

Be open about emotions

Stay busy

Set realistic goals

Be responsible

Avoid complacency

Practice relaxation exercises

Set boundaries with people

Avoid boredom/downtime

Have/get a sense of humor

Manage anger

Avoid self-medication

Be gentle with yourself

Surrender your ideas—go with others' ideas

Be persistent

Sobriety Checklist

The sobriety checklist, which begins on the next page, will help you get started in recovery and track your progress. As you complete each activity, simply place a "√" in the box next to each item completed. Checking the boxes will provide a visual of your actions and progress.

Here is how the Sobriety Checklist is organized (4 pages):

- Page 1: **Recovery Readings** checklist
    - o   Start by reading the Introduction and Chapters 1 and 2 of this book (which you may have already done.)

- Page 2: **12 Step Related Activity** and **Other Recovery Activity** checklists.
    - o   Start these activities as you begin reading Chapter 3.
    - o   Following the order of the items is recommended, but not mandatory. Consistent progress *is* important.
    - o   You can find/review how to accomplish each task by turning to the page number in the right-hand column.

- Page 3: **Meetings, Phone Numbers, and Calls** checklists
    - o   Checklist to track your first 90 meetings
    - o   Checklist to track collection of up to 20 phone contacts
        - ▪   You can enter the numbers into your phone instead of writing them down if you'd like.
        - ▪   Check a box for each number you get.
    - o   Checklist to track your first 90 phone calls

- Page 4: **Sobriety "Chips" & Step-work with Sponsor** √-lists
    - •   Checklist in celebration of your sobriety milestones
    - •   Checklist to track step work you will do with your sponsor

My hope for you is that, by the time you have completed these checklists, you will have put into place a recovery program that will provide the basis for your long-term recovery.

> **Be sure to read the "Detox Warning" on page 14 and take any indicated action. Withdrawal from many drugs can be life threatening, so you want to be sure you aren't putting yourself in danger when you stop using.**

Here is the checklist to track your reading. These readings are very important to understanding your recovery and the actions necessary to attain it. Remember, you will want to begin taking action on the "12 Step Related Activities" checklist on the following page as you read Chapter 3.

√	Recovery Readings	Page Number
	Read Introduction - *Enough Already!*	i-viii
	Read Chapter 1 - *Enough Already!*	1
	Read Chapter 2 - *Enough Already!*	13
	Read Chapter 3 - *Enough Already!*	31
	Read Chapter 4 - *Enough Already!*	39
	Read Chapter 5 - *Enough Already!*	51
	Read Chapter 6 - *Enough Already!*	81
	Read Chapter 7 - *Enough Already!*	107
	Read Chapter 8 - *Enough Already!*	135
	Read Chapter 9 - *Enough Already!*	141
	Read Preface and Forwards - *Big Book*	BB pg. xi-xxiv
	Read Doctor's Opinion - *Big Book*	BB pg. xxxv
	Read Chapter 1 - *Big Book*	BB pg. 1
	Read Chapter 2 - *Big Book*	BB pg. 17
	Read Chapter 3 - *Big Book*	BB pg. 30
	Read Chapter 4 - *Big Book*	BB pg. 44
	Read Chapter 5 - *Big Book*	BB pg. 58
	Read Chapter 6 - *Big Book*	BB pg. 72
	Read Chapter 7 - *Big Book*	BB pg. 89
	Read Chapter 8 - *Big Book*	BB pg. 104
	Read Chapter 9 - *Big Book*	BB pg. 122
	Read Chapter 10 - *Big Book*	BB pg. 136
	Read Chapter 11 - *Big Book*	BB pg. 151
	Read Personal Stories - Part 1 *Big Book*	BB pg. 171
	Read Personal Stories - Part 2 *Big Book*	BB pg. 281
	Read Personal Stories - Part 3 *Big Book*	BB pg. 437
	Read Forward - *12 & 12*	*12 & 12* pg. 15
	Read Step 1 - *12 & 12*	*12 & 12* pg. 21
	Read Step 2 - *12 & 12*	*12 & 12* pg. 25
	Read Step 3 - *12 & 12*	*12 & 12* pg. 34
	Read Step 4 - *12 & 12*	*12 & 12* pg. 42
	Read Steps 5 – 12 *12 & 12*	*12 & 12* pg. 55

Here is the action you will want to take as you read Chapter 3. Remember, the page number in the right-hand column indicates where to find how to accomplish each activity. As you begin going to meetings and making phone calls to your sober support system, you can track them separately on the next page. You can also track your sobriety "chips" and the step work you do with your sponsor on the last page of the checklist.

√	12 Step Related Activity	Page Number
	Called AA, NA, or CA to identify 1st meeting to attend	14-19, 33-36
	Went to 1st meeting (Don't drive under the influence)	14-19, 33-36
	Took "Welcome Chip" (1st mtg. - track chips on pg. 29)	29
	Got phone list at meeting (1st meeting if you can)	34
	Got meeting directory (1st meeting if you can)	34
	Planned weekly meeting schedule (Use the directory)	14-18
	Got "Big Book" (1st week if you can)	22, 34
	Made 1st phone call (Track calls on next page)	21-22
	Went to meeting #2 (Track meetings on next page)	14-18
	Shared at meeting	18
	Started looking for sponsor	19-21
	Purchased *12 & 12* book	23
	Purchased morning meditation book	23
	Develop/start morning recovery routine	46, 87-88, 101, 135
	Took meeting commitment (when opportunity arises)	18
	Shook a newcomer's hand	18
	Got sponsor	19-21
	Did something fun	47
	Went to fellowship after meeting	19

√	Other Recovery Activity	Page #
	Safely dispose of all alcohol, drugs, and paraphernalia	135-136
	Considered professional counseling (See Appendix 2 for referrals)	48, Appx. 2
	Started daily feelings journal	39
	Copied ingredients for recovery	23-24, 80, 135
	Copied trigger list – highlighted top 6 - 8 triggers	75-76, 80, 135
	Copied warning signs – highlighted top 6 - 8 warning signs	79-80, 135
	Added daily review of above 3 copied lists to a.m. recovery routine	80, 135
	Wrote Gratitude List (highly recommended when negativity arises)	61
	Wrote Goodbye Letter	131-133
	Develop/start evening program routine	101-102, 138
	Started exercise program	44-45
	Did something else fun	47
	Went on 12-Step panel	19, 106

√		√		√	MEETINGS	√		√		√	
	#1		#16		#31		#46		#61		#76
	#2		#17		#32		#47		#62		#77
	#3		#18		#33		#48		#63		#78
	#4		#19		#34		#49		#64		#79
	#5		#20		#35		#50		#65		#80
	#6		#21		#36		#51		#66		#81
	#7		#22		#37		#52		#67		#82
	#8		#23		#38		#53		#68		#83
	#9		#24		#39		#54		#69		#84
	#10		#25		#40		#55		#70		#85
	#11		#26		#41		#56		#71		#86
	#12		#27		#42		#57		#72		#87
	#13		#28		#43		#58		#73		#88
	#14		#29		#44		#59		#74		#89
	#15		#30		#45		#60		#75		#90

Check one box for each phone number you get.

√		Contact Name	Phone#'s (optional)	√		Contact Name	Phone #'s optional)
	#1		( )		#11		( )
	#2		( )		#12		( )
	#3		( )		#13		( )
	#4		( )		#14		( )
	#5		( )		#15		( )
	#6		( )		#16		( )
	#7		( )		#17		( )
	#8		( )		#18		( )
	#9		( )		#19		( )
	#10		( )		#20		( )

√		√		√	CALLS	√		√		√	
	#1		#16		#31		#46		#61		#76
	#2		#17		#32		#47		#62		#77
	#3		#18		#33		#48		#63		#78
	#4		#19		#34		#49		#64		#79
	#5		#20		#35		#50		#65		#80
	#6		#21		#36		#51		#66		#81
	#7		#22		#37		#52		#67		#82
	#8		#23		#38		#53		#68		#83
	#9		#24		#39		#54		#69		#84
	#10		#25		#40		#55		#70		#85
	#11		#26		#41		#56		#71		#86
	#12		#27		#42		#57		#72		#87
	#13		#28		#43		#58		#73		#88
	#14		#29		#44		#59		#74		#89
	#15		#30		#45		#60		#75		#90

	"Chips" (a coin, key chain, marble, etc.) are given to group members in celebration of consecutive days without any mind-altering substances. Chips are given at meetings for 30, 60, and 90 days, 6 months, 9 months, one year, and multiple years of sobriety (AKA "birthdays"). Many meetings also acknowledge birthdays by providing a cake with candles and singing "Happy Birthday." "Welcome" chips are also given for newcomers in their first 30 days.

√	Sobriety "Chips"	Pg. 47
	Welcome chip	
	30 day chip	
	60 day chip	
	90 day chip	
	6 month chip	
	9 month chip	
	1-year chip/cake	

HAPPY BIRTHDAY!!!

√	Step-work with Sponsor	√	
	Step 1		Step 7
	Step 2		Step 8
	Step 3		Step 9
	Step 4		Step 10
	Step 5		Step 11
	Step 6		Step 12

For sober coaching and/or online recovery counseling/educational opportunities with Bob Tyler, please visit his website at www.bobtyler.net and hit the "Sober Coaching" tab at the top of the page.

CHAPTER 3
GETTING STARTED

I hope what we have covered thus far regarding the recipe for recovery has furthered the inspiration and hope that caused you to
open this book. If you have a sincere desire for recovery, and are
willing to follow this recipe, you will attain the freedom from drugs
and alcohol that millions of people around the world have enjoyed. If
you have such a desire, hang on to your seat – you're in for the ride of
your life.

Detoxification

Having made the decision for a new life of sobriety, the first thing that
must be considered is whether or not you need a medically supervised
detoxification from whatever you're abusing. If you are addicted to
alcohol, barbiturates, sedatives such as benzodiazapines, GHB, and
some of the newer designer drugs, withdrawal from these can be **life-
threatening**. Additionally, if you are addicted to heroin, morphine,
codeine, Vicodin or other opiates, although not typically life-
threatening, the discomfort associated with withdrawal from these
drugs can become so bad that you may not be able to abstain without
some form of professional help.

There are a couple of different ways to detox in such situations. First,
there is inpatient detox in which you check yourself into a hospital setting where you are monitored by a medical staff and typically given
medication that will decrease the danger associated with detox. Although detox is never completely comfortable, such medication will
usually make it much more tolerable and safe.

Another possibility is an ambulatory (outpatient) detox in which you
see a doctor who prescribes medication on an outpatient basis. Candi-

dates for this type of detox typically need to be highly motivated for recovery. They should also have a support system that will be able to facilitate transportation to and from the doctor's office, since driving is not recommended while taking detox medication. Since detox is only the first part of the recovery process, doctors want to ensure that you'll have a fighting chance at long-term abstinence. Therefore, many doctors who conduct such detox will also want you to be involved in a chemical dependence treatment program.

There are simple ways of determining whether or not you need a medically monitored detox and, if so, whether it should be done on an inpatient or outpatient basis. One way is to simply go see your doctor and let him/her know what and how much you are using so the doctor can determine what level of care, if any, is necessary. Another way is to be assessed at an alcohol or drug treatment center and follow their recommendations. This can be arranged by simply picking up the yellow pages and looking at the listings for "alcohol treatment" or "drug treatment." You can also use the "Treatment Referral Line" and website provided in Appendix 2 near the end of this book. Most treatment centers provide a free assessment and can let you know whether or not you need to be medically detoxed. Such treatment centers will usually provide referrals based on your ability to pay. If you have medical insurance, and have an alcohol or drug detox benefit, the insurance company may pay for all or part of your detoxification. Many treatment centers are willing to check your benefits for you. However, you can check the benefits yourself by calling the number on your insurance card. If you do not have insurance or other financial means to pay for your treatment, you will likely be referred to a county-funded program. In many parts of the country, availability is sometimes difficult because they are often full. If you are persistent and determined to succeed, entry into one of these programs can be accomplished. If it has been determined that you need a medical detox, and are having difficulty in finding a detox center you can afford, the National Counsel on Alcoholism and Drug Dependence (NCADD) is a very good referral resource that can aid you in finding treatment. Simply look in the phone book or call information to get the phone number of the local NCADD. Again, you can also use the "Treatment Referral Line" and website provided in Appendix 2 near the end of this book.

I highly recommend, whether detox is needed or not, that you enter a chemical dependence rehabilitation program. This can be done in an inpatient or outpatient setting. It gives you a good head start on your recovery because such centers provide much education and support in your early recovery. Participating in treatment with others who have had similar struggles with addiction, makes you realize you are not alone. You also come away with a strong support system of peers with whom you have gone through treatment. Additionally, you will likely become connected to the 12-Step meetings the treatment center has you attend. If you decide to try recovery without the formal treatment that follows detox, make a commitment to yourself to pursue formal treatment if you continue to relapse without it (if needed, please see "Treatment Referral Line" in Appendix 2.)

In summary, get a consultation from a physician, or get a free assessment at a treatment center to find out whether or not you need a medical detox. If you do, ask for a referral based on your ability to pay and pursue it. Again, whether or not you need such a detox, I do recommend getting formal chemical dependence treatment if you have the means to do so. If you would like to get such treatment, ask for a referral based on your ability to pay or call your local NCADD. Even if you are only able to get on a waiting list, you may want to do it so that you can eventually go to formal treatment if you continue to relapse.

Working a 12-Step Program

Whether or not you have decided to pursue a formal treatment program, it is now time to get started with 12-Step meeting attendance. If you do not know where to find meetings, simply look in the white pages of your local telephone book (I just looked in my local phone book and found Alcoholics Anonymous, Narcotics Anonymous, and Cocaine Anonymous). If you cannot find such programs in the white pages, you should be able to find the number for the nearest NCADD there. You might also find the listing in the yellow pages under "Alcohol Treatment" or "Drug Treatment." If you don't succeed in finding 12-Step programs in this way, you can always call a treatment center in your area, which can also be found in the yellow page listings. Simply ask for the telephone number of your 12-Step program of choice. When you call the 12-Step program, ask the person who answers the phone where the 12-Step meetings are in your area. Meetings in many areas are held at multiple locations every day of the week. You can also refer to Appendix 2 for the national offices of 12 Step programs.

I stand firm on my recommendation to attend 90 meetings in 90 days for reasons I have already outlined. If you feel you are not ready for this kind of a commitment to your recovery, begin attending anyway. You may come to find that my suggestion is not all that outlandish at all and will eventually build up to that level of attendance. If going to less meetings than "90 in 90" is the route you choose to take, make a firm commitment to yourself that if you continue to relapse, you will take my suggestion and begin attending daily. Do not engage in the insanity of many people who have gone before you – trying the same thing over and over again and expecting different results.

Remember, it is best to get to the meeting a little early as it enhances your chances of getting to know people before the meeting. This will help you to begin building your sober support system – one of the main objectives in attending meetings. I suggest you pick up three things at that first meeting. First, you want to get a meeting directory for your area. Most meetings will have either a directory for your immediate area (often free of charge), or a directory for a larger area that typically costs about a dollar and a half. Next, most meetings also have a phone list which you'll want to get. This way, you'll have numbers to call if you feel like using or need to talk to someone who understands what new people in recovery experience. Finally, pick up the book that contains the program of recovery for AA, NA, or CA. The book title is the same as the name of the fellowship you are attending – *Alcoholics Anonymous, Narcotics Anonymous, or Cocaine Anonymous.* Such books are typically in the neighborhood of five to ten dollars depending on the area you live in. If you cannot afford one right away, most meetings will provide one if you promise to pay later. You might also want to purchase the *12 and 12* to aid you with step work, and a morning meditation book so you can start each day focused on recovery.

As mentioned earlier, it is best to attend the same meetings each week, as this will eventually make you feel more at home when you attend. This will also enable you to make friends at such meetings. If you don't particularly care for a given meeting, then find another one for that day of the week and attend it weekly. Shop around. There are many different types of meetings in various types of settings. I found that meetings held in church halls were most comfortable for me. I encourage you to find what is most comfortable for you and seek such meetings out.

Don't be discouraged if none of the meetings feel very comfortable for you. This is common for someone in early recovery and it takes some getting used to hearing people talk so openly about things you might never

> Don't be discouraged if none of the meetings feel very comfortable for you.

have dreamed of sharing in the past. Just keep attending, even if it feels uncomfortable, and you will eventually achieve a level of comfort in being there. I implore you not to make the mistake many others have in the past by judging how the meetings make you feel in the early going and making the decision that it can't possibly work for you. It *will* work if you give it a chance. Resist the negativity that may arise for you at the meetings and remember that you don't know the first thing about recovery so how would you know what is helpful. You are doing this not because you think it is a good idea, but because people who know much more than you about staying sober are suggesting it.

I had some initial difficulty myself with such meetings. One of my biggest problems was that I would go into a meeting focused on what it had to offer me. If I didn't feel like I got anything out of the meeting, I would walk away resentful and wondering if I was doing the right thing. It was suggested to me that, instead of going to the meeting looking for what I could take from it, I should focus on what I could bring to the meeting with my presence. With this attitude, I was never disappointed.

At speaker meetings, I often found myself sizing up the speaker in an attempt to determine whether or not the speaker deserved to be at the podium. I often came to the conclusion that the person had nothing to offer me. Consequently, I would ignore what the person had to say and feel that I wasted my time at that meeting. It was suggested to me that, in such a situation, I listen intently for the one piece of information the person might have to offer me. This is based on the idea that for each sobriety pitch I hear, there is only a small percentage of the talk I will actually take with me and keep for the long-term – even if I was very interested in hearing what the person had to say. This suggestion aided me in staying focused no matter who was speaking.

It is also helpful to focus on the similarities you have with others in the group, rather than the differences. It is easy to look at the differences between yourself and others at the meetings and to make a case for why you shouldn't be there. It is common for people to refer to our problem as "terminal uniqueness." This is due to the fact that many people die from this disease because they stay focused on how unique their case is and discount their potential for recovery in the midst of people who can't possibly understand. Whether you know it or not, they *do* understand and have the same difficulty you do in tolerating the emotion arising from difficult circumstances. Focusing on the similarities is truly in your control and I encourage you to begin doing that now.

When you feel ready, begin asking for the phone numbers of people you may have connected with at the meeting. It is vital that you eventually do this so you will have people to call when you need support through the difficult times early sobriety typically poses. You should also be keeping your eyes and ears open for a potential sponsor who can also support you through the difficult times, and who can help you in working the steps. Also, when your particular meetings offer opportunities for commitments, volunteer for one of them as this will also increase your visibility at meetings and people will get to know you better. Meeting commitments will also help you to get to meetings when you don't feel like going because people are depending on you to be there.

Also, when you feel ready, begin sharing at meetings. This is probably the best way to break the barrier that gets in the way of your meeting people. You will be amazed at the response you get from even the most simple and/or brief share. It also allows you to start getting some of the skeletons out of your closet by sharing your own difficulties with alcohol or drug use.

Do not allow yourself to go much longer than 30 days without choosing a sponsor. The sooner you get one, the sooner you will be able to start working the steps. When you find a sponsor, ask him or her if it is okay to call every day. If it is (and it should be or you may have picked the wrong sponsor), take my suggestion and do so. Also tell your sponsor that you are ready to work the steps as soon as possible. (Refer back to Chapter 2 for tips on finding a sponsor.)

I want to recommend telling those around you what you are doing, except in situations which might be damaging to you, such as, telling your boss if he or she does not already know what is happening. Telling those around you increases your accountability. If everyone knows you are trying to stay sober, it is much harder to drink or use. Along with the resulting decrease in maneuverability of your disease, this will also prompt others to be supportive of your decision to stop by not offering you alcohol or drugs and not drinking or using around you. The following chapter includes some additional ingredients that are vital to recovery.

CHAPTER 4
MORE INGREDIENTS FOR RECOVERY

Journal writing is a valuable tool in recovery because it allows you to process your feelings on paper. When in your addiction, you use chemicals to repress your feelings. When getting sober, you are flooded by such repressed feelings and this can be very overwhelming. Without appropriate outlets for such feelings, you will eventually become so consumed by them that returning to the use of chemicals will feel like your only alternative. So, along with sharing your feelings with your sponsor, sober peers, and at meetings, you can also process them on paper.

Your feelings can often become very confusing and you might not have the ability to sort them out simply by leaving them in your head. When you get the feelings on paper, and read them back to yourself, you gain new insight into the feelings. There is also a tendency to be honest when writing. Again, by reading what is written, you gain significant insight into what is really happening with you. For example, if you happened to be particularly angry on a given day, you can explore such anger by writing about it. Simply begin writing about your anger and then exploring on paper why you are so angry. You may often come to the conclusion that your anger is the result of masking other uncomfortable feelings such as fear, shame, or sadness. Thus, you find out that your anger is secondary to other emotions. You can then experience the underlying emotions while processing them on paper and, as a result, gain some emotional growth and maturity. I recommend journaling for 10 minutes every day, whether or not you feel the need to.

Developing a spiritual program is very important in recovery, as we will see in Chapter 6. Please, do not confuse a spiritual program with a religious program. In what is referred to as religion, people engage in some form of worship of a *particular* God. Examples of religion include Christianity, Judaism, Hinduism, Islam, and Buddhism, among others. Step 2 of AA reads: "Came to believe that a Power greater than ourselves could restore us to sanity" (Alcoholics Anonymous, 2001, p. 59). For a given individual, this "Higher Power" can be the God they may have found through a particular religion, or a Higher Power of his or her own personal understanding. Although the founders of AA were influenced by the Christian religion, they realized after writing the steps that some people may be turned off by a program that refers to a particular religion. As a result, the words in Step 3 now read: "…turn our will and our lives over to the care of God *as we understood Him*" (Alcoholics Anonymous, 2001, p. 59). This opens the program up to everyone and the Higher Power can be anything the addict chooses. The only requirement is that the addict believes it is strong enough to help with what the addict has failed miserably at – staying sober.

Developing a spiritual program may include **prayer, meditation,** and reading spiritual or personal religious material. Many in the program make a distinction between prayer and meditation with which I agree: prayer is talking to God, and meditation is listening to God.

Avoiding using/drinking people and places in early recovery is very important due to the obvious danger such situations pose. You have absolutely no business being around alcohol and/or drugs of any type for at least the first few months of sobriety! I acknowledge this might seem unreasonable since alcohol and drugs permeate our society. A common response to this suggestion is, "What do I need to do, live in a closet the rest of my life?" These same people go against the suggestion and may have some success at staying sober at first. However, in almost every case, they eventually break down and drink again. Remember, if you hang around a barbershop long enough, you'll eventually get a haircut!

> You have absolutely no business being around alcohol and/or drugs of any type for at least the first few months of sobriety!

Clients who relapse due to such carelessness often say that "It did not bother me at all" or "I was even repulsed by seeing it," and they can't understand why they drank again. One reason might be that there is a subconscious process going on in which the alcoholic feels left out because others appear to be having a good time. Perhaps they feel isolated or different from everyone else. What is very important to understand here is that we often don't know when or why a relapse might strike.

Often in early recovery, when the initial crisis that brings addicts or alcoholics into treatment is over, a feeling of overconfidence and complacency sets in. This is often called the "Pink Cloud." They have no desire to drink and feel much of this stuff is merely "overkill." This way of thinking is extremely dangerous and I hope my bringing it to your attention will help you to avoid it. In the Big Book of AA, it states, "The alcoholic at certain times has no effective mental defense against the first drink" (Alcoholics Anonymous 2001, p. 43). We will *all* have such times. If one of these times happens and you are in a drinking or using situation, the combination spells relapse. Therefore, if you minimize how often you are in such situations, you lessen the chance for such a lethal combination to occur. No matter how confident you might be about not taking that first drink, **you are still at risk!**

Avoiding isolation is important because we have proven we cannot do this thing alone. Many alcoholics and addicts in the program speak of what they call: "The Committee." This committee is in your head, is typically very negative, and tells you all the reasons why it is a good idea for you to drink or use. When you isolate, you are allowing this committee to provide you with lethal lies without interruption. Another program saying is this: "When you are alone in your head, you are in a bad neighborhood." So it is vital that we go to a lot of meetings, hang out with recovering people, and make plenty of phone calls so the committee can be interrupted on a regular basis.

> "The alcoholic at certain times has no effective mental defense against the first drink" (Alcoholics Anonymous, 1976, p. 43).

Setting boundaries with using friends

When I was in the treatment center where I started my sobriety, I was told I had to get rid of all the so-called friends I used to drink and use with. This was very difficult for me to accept. I felt that some of the people I used with were more than just using buddies. In fact, some of these friends wanted me to get sober way before I wanted me to get sober. This was especially apparent when I showed up at a poker game on the third day of a binge with a bag full of cocaine. I looked like something the cat dragged in and my friends shared with me they felt I better get some help. Therefore, I felt they would be very supportive of my recovery if I kept them in my life. However, I had taken nearly every suggestion that was given me in early recovery and I was scared to make the exception here.

With the help of my counselors and sponsor, I was able to recognize I was in no position to make a rational decision regarding which of these people would, in fact, be supportive of my recovery. This is because I was emotionally attached to them. I, therefore, agreed to stay away from all such people for about the first six months of my recovery. This would allow me to, in effect, emotionally "detox" from them so I would be more capable of making a rational decision regarding who should remain in my life.

Regarding most of these people, it was clear to me that I needed to end the relationship and grieve the loss. However, there were a handful of them whom I felt could probably remain in my life. I called these people to let them know that I was going to have to do my own thing so they won't be hearing from me for a while. I also told them that when the time was right, I would be contacting them so we might get together.

After about six months, and having built a solid foundation of sobriety, I was able to make rational decisions regarding whom I thought would be supportive of my sobriety. This period of time also allowed me to determine what boundaries I would need to set with these guys if we were to continue our friendships. These boundaries were based on what triggers were still in effect in my life. There were only a handful of guys I felt could remain in my life and my initial telephone call to them went something like this:

"Hi Mike. Thanks for giving me the space I needed to pursue my recovery. As you might imagine, my sobriety is very important to me. Even though we used together in the past, I need you to be 100% supportive of my sobriety in order for us to continue our friendship. This is how you can be supportive of me. First, I don't mind if you drink beer around me, but I would be too uncomfortable if I saw you drinking whiskey. Second, if we get together and you and the guys want to smoke a joint, please warn me so either you guys or I can leave the room so I don't have to smell it. Finally, in regards to cocaine, I can't see you using it, or be around you when you're on it – I don't want to hear anything about it. My sobriety is so important to me that if you cross any of these boundaries, I will consider it a threat to my life and we can no longer be friends."

It was very uncomfortable making rules that our friendship was contingent upon, but it was absolutely necessary. The response I got from these guys was 100% supportive and they have always kept these commitments to me. Had they balked at these boundaries, it would have been a clear message that they did not care enough about me to be my friends. An important note here is that, even though I set such boundaries, I still had to take responsibility for my own sobriety. I needed to realize that if they drank too much, they might not remember the promises they made to me. Therefore, I needed to use my best judgment and leave if they should drink too much. Additionally, if they are drinking excessively, I really have no business being there in the first place because that's not what I'm about anymore. I get satisfaction out of reality-based activities today – not those that are surrounded by mind-altering substances.

Honesty is one of the most important aspects of recovery. The Big Book calls for "rigorous honesty" and, at the start of chapter five, its importance is stressed. In my experience as a counselor, I can make this statement with all confidence: If you are dishonest in recovery, you will *not* stay sober. Such dishonesty goes

> If you are dishonest in recovery, you will *not* stay sober.

beyond merely lying. It includes withholding the truth, living a dishonest lifestyle, and not being open and truthful about your feelings. For example, if you relapse and don't tell anyone about it, you will not get the help you need. If you are engaging in illegal activity or cheating on your wife or husband, you are working against what you are trying to achieve in your new life.

Many in the program identify themselves as "liars, cheats and thieves" and, if you have any of these characteristics, you must change in order to be comfortable in your own skin. Since alcoholics and addicts are such sensitive people, you simply cannot engage in such behavior because it eventually eats away at you and relapse inevitably occurs.

I have seen this happen to many people since I've been in recovery and exceptions are rare. I can remember observing the behavior of a man who had 11 years of sobriety and was cheating on his wife. I was amazed that this person was staying sober while living this secret life. Much to my disappointment, this man did eventually relapse. This validated everything I know about the importance of honesty in all aspects of our lives.

I sometimes found it difficult sharing honestly at meetings when I was having a difficult time dealing with life on life's terms. My ego told me that I shouldn't have such difficult times when I had so much sobriety time. However, if I didn't allow myself to be honest in such situations, how was I going to get the help I needed? How was someone to reach out to me if they didn't know I needed help? God knows I certainly needed help because I failed miserably, and often still do, in solving my own problems.

Exercise is also a valuable tool for recovery. When you exercise, you feel physically better due to being more fit and healthy. This is also due to the fact that, when you exercise, your brain releases natural opiate-like substances called endorphins that give you a natural sense of well-being. You also tend to feel better psychologically when you feel good physically. Additionally, there is a direct psychological benefit due to the good feeling you get from taking good care of yourself. When you feel good physically and psychologically, there is a tendency to feel less stress. And the less stress you have, the less likely it is that you will relapse. Exercise as used above can be viewed as a preventative maintenance tool against relapse. However, it can also be used as a tool against relapse when an active craving for drugs or alcohol strikes. **Be sure to consult a physician regarding any physical limitations you might have that would limit your ability to engage in an exercise program.**

*In my own recovery, when I got a craving I had three favorite tools I used: I said a prayer to my Higher Power; I called my sponsor or another member of my sober support system; and **I thought the relapse through** to its logical ending. One day I got a craving and engaged in all three of the above interventions. However, a minor craving persisted. I don't know what compelled me, but I decided to run out of the house and around the block. I did so at a very fast pace. When I returned home, my heart was beating fast, my blood was flowing, and I was breathing heavily. I suddenly realized that, miraculously, the craving was completely gone!*

Adequate sleep is essential in recovery because, when tired, you have increased irritability and are not thinking at full capacity. Recovery is so tenuous that you need to remain alert to the possibility of relapse at all times. Additionally, just as you feel physically and psychologically better when you exercise, the same holds true for having adequate rest.

Proper diet is also important due to the fact that eating is probably not a priority in the midst of your disease. Consequently, you deplete your body of essential nutrients needed for health and well-being. By eating a balanced diet, you replace such nutrients. A word of warning regarding food intake: I have seen many people use food to anesthetize feelings instead of drugs or alcohol. So watch for overeating and/or eating unhealthy foods. If you are an alcoholic, you must also be aware of the possibility of becoming addicted to sugar. As part of the metabolization process, alcohol is eventually broken down into a sugar in your body. When you stop drinking, your body craves the missing sugar. In fact, a portion of the Big Book quotes a doctor who stated, "…occasionally in the night a vague craving arose which would be satisfied by candy" (*Alcoholics Anonymous*, 2001, p.134). On occasion this is probably fine, as long as it is not done excessively.

Thinking positive thoughts helps rescue you from the negativity that drives many addicts to relapse. Negativity is a very common trait among the addicted and prevents openness, willingness, and teachability. This is especially detrimental in early recovery when you are receiving suggestions for new ways of thinking and behaving. Negativity will reject any new idea that comes your way. I am a firm believer that a positive can be found in any negative if you look hard enough. And let's face it, who do you think is going to be the happier person: the one who is positive or the one who is negative?

Structure your life so you have a minimum of time alone with no activity. Structure provides activities in your daily living so you know what you'll be doing from one moment to the next. If you leave a couple hours of your day open in early recovery, your sick mind will be allowed to think up some unhealthy way of filling the time. This does not mean that you shouldn't have any time alone – we all need that. However, it does mean that what we do with that time should be planned ahead to avoid unhealthy diversion. It is always a good idea to try to plan to do something with another person – preferably with someone in recovery. This creates accountability and prevents loneliness.

A good way to start your day, along with morning meditation and prayer, is to review your day to determine if you have left open any extended period of time. If you have, devise a plan to fill that time constructively. A great time filler is to get a job or enroll in school. In this way, large chunks of time are accounted for in productive activity.

In my early sobriety, I was working full time and attending meetings daily. So I would go to work, go home for dinner, and head out to a meeting. Consequently, the challenge of how to fill my time was reduced to weekends only. This was difficult and I felt like all I was doing was working and going to meetings. In hindsight, this was the best thing for me in early recovery because I knew how just about every hour would be spent each day. This was also difficult for my wife because I was not able to spend much time with her. What made it easier for both of us was remembering that this level of program activity would be temporary, and that it was a worthwhile investment in attaining a new life. It really paid dividends.

Having fun is an often overlooked, but crucial element of recovery. If you don't take the time to have fun in sobriety, your addicted mind will tell you, "Heck, at least when I was out there using I had a little fun." This leads to resentment about your recovery and eventually to relapse. **Developing hobbies**, or re-engaging in old ones, is a good way to create fun in your life. If you are having difficulty coming up with ideas on how to have fun in sobriety, think back to your pre-using days about what you enjoyed doing. Asking people with time in sobriety what they do for fun will also be helpful. If you are in a treatment program, their alumni association will likely have sober activities to show you that fun can be had in sobriety.

"Thinking it through" is very important when a craving hits. As I stated above, it is one of my favorite tools in recovery. Craving typically results from focusing on how good that first hit, drink, or pill will be. Thinking the using episode through to its logical ending aids you in focusing on the negatives of using, rather than the positives. This is done by envisioning what will happen after that first drink or fix, and what happens after that, etc., until you get to the back end of the relapse when you have all the consequences and regrets. This focus on the negative consequences aids in squelching your craving.

Being persistent in your program of recovery involves keeping your enthusiasm for sobriety to the point that you continue engaging in the program activity that has aided you in attaining sobriety. It is very easy to become overconfident and complacent. This results in the tendency to take your sobriety for granted. In my experience, an extremely high percentage of relapses occur in this way. Do not allow the negativity and lack of enthusiasm that you might see in others to rub off on you. Migrate to those who share your enthusiasm and persistence. If you feel like you lack enthusiasm at any point in your sobriety, hang out with those who have it. They will have a much better influence on you than someone who might validate your negativity and lack of enthusiasm. As many in 12-Step programs say: "**Stick with the winners**."

Creating a sobriety plan is especially important when you are anticipating exposure to triggers and believe your sobriety might be in danger. In very early sobriety, it is highly recommended not to get into such situations. As will be discussed in the next chapter, at some point in your sobriety you will begin to create a sobriety plan that will enable exposure to some triggers. This is part of the trigger recovery process.

Good hygiene – Many with our disease develop an "I don't give a damn" attitude. Self-care gives you a very clear message that you are beginning to "give a damn" about yourself. This becomes reflected in other behavior as well. However, if you look in the mirror and look like crap, it can be depressing and gives you the message that you are worthless, inferior, and that you still don't give a hoot about anything. This attitude extends to recovery as it leads to not caring about sobriety either – an attitude that can be deadly.

Professional counseling is a very good adjunct to working a 12-Step program and I highly recommend it if you can afford it. It is essential that you select a counselor that has experience in working with alcoholics and addicts and one who will be supportive of your 12-Step program. For most of the first year of my sobriety, it really helped to receive some direct feedback from a knowledgeable counselor.

Taking direction, as I mentioned at the start of this book, will be the determining factor of whether you get sober or not. As many in the 12-Step programs say, "Your best thinking got you here." Therefore, it is a probably a good idea to trust suggestions from other people, namely, those who have had some success in sobriety.

Avoiding other compulsive behaviors is important because such behavior threatens your sobriety due to the development of cross-addiction. Cross-addiction results because there are similar patterns involved in other compulsive behaviors, such as: running from emotions, dishonesty, and leading a double life. If you continue to run from emotion through the use of such compulsive behavior, you are not really recovering because you are simply switching addictions. Additionally, since your cross-addictive behaviors are similar to your old using patterns, they act as triggers to relapse on your substance of choice.

Sober living homes are available for recovering people to live together and remain focused on a common purpose – staying sober. In most sober living homes, you will share a room with one or more recovering people in a structured environment, which can include curfews and meeting requirements – among other things. People in recovery typically manage such homes and the cost is usually between $300 and $800 monthly depending on the area, the condition of the home, and the structure provided. Sober living is particularly encouraged for recovering people who live alone or in an unsupportive environment. If you fall into this category, and feel this is not necessary for you, you may want to make a commitment to yourself that if you relapse, you will enter one for at least 30 – 60 days.

Vigorously using these tools, along with those discussed in Chapter 2, are crucial to successful recovery. Remember to make a copy of the master list of the ingredients for recovery that can be found at the end of Chapter 2. I realize that viewing this extensive list might seem overwhelming. However, if you view each item individually rather than as a whole, it will be much easier to digest. You do not need to be perfect in recovery. You will gradually incorporate more of the ingredients as you progress in your program. View this list daily to remind you of what you are working toward. This stuff really works and, if you haven't already done so, I encourage you to start the process of getting your life back. Now that we've explored the foundation for recovery, we can look at the keys to relapse prevention.

CHAPTER 5
RELAPSE PREVENTION

When I was approximately 30 days sober, I read an article that changed the course of my recovery. It was called "Cocaine Craving and Relapse" and was printed in *Sober Times: The Recovery Magazine* in early 1989. The article was written by one of the most renowned and knowledgeable relapse preventionists in the world – Terence Gorski. I benefited from this article as much as any information I received while in treatment. The insight and knowledge I gained has compelled me to pass it on to patients and colleagues ever since. If you are not a cocaine addict, don't allow the title of the article to sway your attention – it is just as applicable to any drug of choice.

In the fall of 1999, I had the honor of meeting Mr. Gorski when he spoke at the annual conference of CAADAC (California Association of Alcoholism and Drug Abuse Counselors). I was awed at the opportunity of hearing one of my idols speak in person. I shook his hand at the end of the talk and shared with him what an impact his information has had on my life and career.

Later that night, I was heading for my hotel room across the street, and there came Mr. Gorski walking down the street. Once again, I extended my hand to him and elaborated on the influence he has had on me. I shared about my relapse prevention lecture series, which is largely based on his information that was published a decade prior. He appeared genuinely thrilled that someone was using his information in this way. We talked about many other issues in recovery as well. The next thing we knew, an hour and a half had passed as we spoke at that Sacramento intersection. It was truly one of the thrills of my life. It also gave me great pleasure to have him validate what I was doing. To Mr. Gorski, I am eternally grateful.

So now it is time for me to pass it on to you. This section will, most assuredly, help you deal with craving and minimize its occurrence. The information that follows is based on the article mentioned above, and I have added some of my own personal and professional experience with it.

Craving and Relapse

We will start by exploring "The Craving Cycle" as outlined by Terence Gorski. It consists of:

> Obsession
> Compulsion
> Physical craving
> Drug-seeking behavior (Gorski, 1989)

As a craving "cycle," it typically starts with obsession, moves into compulsion and, finally, into physical craving and drug-seeking behavior. As you will see below, each stage in the craving cycle moves the person increasingly closer to relapse. A brief definition of each of these elements of the craving cycle follows:

Obsession

Obsession is "the inability to stop thinking about the alcohol and drug use." Such a thought is very strong and persistent (Gorski, 1988). It usually starts as a mild thought of using and, if left to run its course, it becomes all encompassing and is characterized by the inability to think about anything else. Therefore, it is very important to intervene on an obsessive thought of using or it will "quickly turn into a compulsion" (Gorski, 2001).

Compulsion

While obsession is a thinking state, "a compulsion is an emotional state that is marked by an urge or desire to use alcohol or drugs" (Gorski, 1988). "When compulsion is activated the person begins experiencing an overwhelming urge to use the drug…" (Gorski, 2001). Since it is an emotional state, you are unable to think rationally. Have you ever made a decision based on emotion that didn't turn out so well? This is what a compulsion causes you to do. You are so emotionally involved that using actually appears to be a good decision. Once a compulsion hits, you are usually unable to make rational sense of it without the assistance of another

> Once a compulsion hits, you are usually unable to make rational sense of it without the assistance of another recovering addict.

recovering addict. As with obsession, it is important to intervene on a compulsion before it gets too strong because you will eventually be rendered unable to use the tools of recovery to deal with it.

Physical Craving

If a compulsion is left uninterrupted, it will eventually "merge into full blown physical craving" (Gorski, 2001). In physical craving, your body is actually asking for the drug of choice. "It is a physical need or tissue hunger for a drug that is caused by brain chemistry imbalances" (Gorski, 1988). *In my disease, when a physical craving became extremely strong, I would actually lose control of bodily functions and would often have to run to the restroom. It is as if my brain was preparing my body for the incoming drugs or alcohol.*

Physical craving also occurs in early sobriety independent of the cycle of craving. When you use drugs or alcohol, you are actually pumping poison into your body. The body compensates for the presence of this poison by actually changing into a transformed state. The more drugs and alcohol you use, the more your body must change to survive. When you stop using, the body cannot survive in this transformed state without the poison, so it must adjust back to its normal state in order to survive. The problem is that the process of changing from its transformed state to its normal state is painful. Therefore, your body begs for more drugs so it can stay comfortable and avoid the pain of changing back to normal. This process of the body changing back to normal is known as withdrawal and, as stated earlier, with some drugs, such as: alcohol, barbiturates, benzodiazapines, GHB, and some of the newer designer drugs, such withdrawal can be painful, cause seizures and hallucinations, and can even be deadly. Withdrawal from opiates like heroin, morphine, and codeine can also be extremely painful. Also stated earlier, it is essential that you consult a physician or have an assessment at a treatment center to determine if you need a medically supervised detoxification.

Drug Seeking Behavior

Eventually, if left untouched, the craving will arrive at this final and most dangerous stage. Drug seeking behavior is just that – it is the action you take to seek out your drug of choice. You "begin to cruise old neighborhoods, talk with old drug-using friends, and go to bars and other places where (alcohol or drugs are) used" (Gorski, 2001). It is important to realize that it is typically "ritualized, habitual behavior" (Gorski, 1988). You often don't even realize you are doing it. You might have a very good reason in your head to go visit George, but George was a using buddy. You might also have rationalized why you are driving down a certain street, but that is where your drug dealer hung out. You might think it's a good idea to go see some old friend at a bar, but it was your favorite watering hole. The reality is that these are all drug-seeking behaviors that often lead to relapse.

More About the Craving Cycle

There are two things you need to know about the craving cycle. First, it occurs at some point for all alcoholics and addicts. No matter how much you got your butt kicked by the disease before you began pursuing sobriety, you will at some point experience craving. Often times, it does not occur right away. You might think this is a good thing, however, it can be quite dangerous. It can lull you into a false sense of security and you might be unprepared when craving strikes. In fact, if you are having many cravings in early sobriety, you will actually have an advantage if you can stay sober. The experience of utilizing the tools of recovery to successfully deal with cravings prepares you for the next time the phenomenon hits.

The other thing that is known about craving is that it always precedes relapse. You don't find yourself walking down the street, tripping over the curb, with a bottle dropping from the sky into your mouth. You will first stop at the craving cycle by thinking about it, becoming emotional about it, your body will start asking for it, and you will eventually seek it out. The facts that craving happens to all alcoholics/addicts, and it always precedes relapse, should tell you that the craving cycle is a very dangerous place that should be avoided as much as possible.

In many alcohol and drug treatment centers, the primary focus is on teaching patients what to do when craving hits. Many of these tools are found in Chapters 2 and 4 of this book. Unfortunately, many centers neglect to teach people how to avoid falling into the craving cycle in the first place. In the next few pages we will do just that – learn how to minimize the frequency of entering the craving cycle. We will accomplish this by focusing on what are called *set-up behaviors* and *trigger events*, two criteria that contribute to the craving cycle. By utilizing this information, you will significantly reduce the frequency of entering it. The fewer set-up behaviors you have, the less often you will end up in the craving cycle. Likewise, if you are aware of your relapse triggers, you will be able to avoid many of them and experience the craving cycle less frequently. This information will also help in identifying the cause of your entrance into the craving cycle so you can deal with it more effectively.

Set-up Behaviors

Set-up behaviors are things that you do to set yourself up for craving. Let us take a look at these behaviors which Gorski (1989) has identified and organized into three categories:

Physical Set-ups
Psychological Set-ups
Social Set-ups

Physical Set-ups

One physical set-up Gorski emphasizes is <u>poor diet.</u> We get so deep into our disease that we tend to "become malnourished or undernourished" (Gorski, 1989). Increasingly more addiction professionals are focusing on the importance of diet in recovery. You need to rebuild your ravaged body which has been torn down by the disease. Additionally, when you eat right, you feel better physically. A natural result of this is you feel better emotionally, decreasing your need to escape to the craving cycle. Furthermore, eating right has a direct psychological effect because a good feeling results from finally taking care of yourself.

Another physical set-up that Gorski speaks of is <u>lack of exercise.</u> "We know that aerobic exercise reduces the intensity of craving experiences... it is one of the few protections we have against craving, especially in the first six to nine months of recovery" (Gorski, 1989). Exercise can be seen as a preventative maintenance measure against craving. Gorski cites the body's natural opiate-like substances (endorphins) in the brain that are released into the body when you exercise. As stated in Chapter 4, endorphins are your body's natural painkillers and they make you feel good. So if you exercise regularly, they are being released on a regular basis leading to a greater sense of well-being. Additionally, when you exercise, you feel physically better due to being more healthy and fit. As with eating right, when you feel physically better, you have a tendency to also feel better psychologically and, therefore, have less need to escape to the craving cycle. Further, there is a direct psychological benefit due to the good feeling you get from finally taking care of yourself. As stated previously, exercise can also be used as a tool against relapse when an active craving for drugs or alcohol hits.

The final physical set-up Gorski presents is <u>poor stress management.</u> "When we do not manage stress in recovery, we increase our risk of a craving because we become stress-sensitive" (Gorski, 1989). Since addicts have a tendency to be ultra-sensitive, daily living can be very stressful. One incident bothers us, then another, and the stress begins to build. Eventually, someone might say or do something that normally wouldn't bother us, and we suddenly blow-up at them. Since anger is one of the leading causes of relapse, we cannot afford to allow our stress to build to that point. Therefore, people in recovery need to learn how to manage each stressful event as it comes by working the tools of recovery. Later in the book, you will learn some relaxation techniques you will find useful in managing your stress.

Psychological Set-ups

When I originally read Gorski's *Cocaine Craving and Relapse* article, it was this section on psychological set-ups, which was of particular value to me. I totally set myself up psychologically for relapse over many years of trying to stop using on my own and in early sobriety. It was life-saving information to me and I hope it impacts you in the same way.

Euphoric Recall

"When we are in euphoric recall, we remember and exaggerate pleasurable memories of past chemical use episodes. Then we block or repress our bad memories of drug use or deny the pain associated with them" (Gorski, 1989). This makes sense because, when you start into the craving cycle, you are not thinking about how bad it will be – you are thinking about how good the first drink, hit, or pill will be. The most important part of this section on set-up behaviors is this: If you can recognize when you are engaging in them, you can take appropriate action and, thus, deter entry into the craving cycle. So if you can recognize that you're focusing on the positive aspects of using, you can simply begin focusing on the negative aspects. It is often just that simple.

In personal use of this strategy, I have found that the sooner I recognize my euphoric recall, the easier it is to shift my focus. If it continues unnoticed by me for any significant period of time, it becomes difficult to simply switch my thoughts from the positives of using to the negatives. At such times, I utilize one of my favorite tools of recovery that I mentioned earlier – "thinking the using episode through." This is a systematic way of moving my thoughts from the positives to the negatives of using – from romancing to reality. What follows is an example of thinking it through – a night in the life of Bob, the addict:

First let me set the scene by telling you how bad my disease had gotten during the period I am going to describe. Since my wife, Robin, was working nights, I was able to use drugs after she went to work without being hassled. I would come home and have dinner with her before she left, all the while knowing I would deceitfully get loaded as soon as she went out the door. I would usually bring home enough cocaine to last me until about midnight so I could get a decent night's sleep, despite the fact that I had proven to myself hundreds of times that I could not succeed with this plan. So I would finish what I had and end up driving from San Gabriel (we had done a geographic change a year earlier thinking we could move away from the problem) down to Hawthorne to pick up some more stash. I then proceeded to use all night.

When the rooster across the street crowed at dawn, it signified to me the using episode was ending and I would think to myself, "You idiot! You did it again." I then started the process of cleaning up any evidence of use before Robin returned from work. Right before she returned home, I would go upstairs into the bedroom, wipe off my sweat, push the pillow up tightly against my eyes to create the illusion I had been sleeping all night, and pretend I was asleep as she walked into the bedroom. She would get ready for bed (often with much suspicion I'm sure), lie down next to me, and conveniently put her hand on my chest. My heart would be racing and she would know I was using. I would play this off by telling her I must have had a bad dream and proceed to get up and get ready for work.

The following "think it through" scenario is not extraordinary. It is simply typical of what happened every time I used cocaine. It was New Year's Eve, 1987 – approximately 11 months before I got sober. Robin had to work that night, but I very much wanted to go to our annual New Year's Eve party with all our friends. I told her that I only had $50 and would only use that much cocaine and return home safely by 1:00 am. I fully believed that I could accomplish this. She halfheartedly agreed and I went to the party.

I arrived there and bought $50 worth of cocaine and proceeded to get high very innocently with my friends. This cocaine did not last me long and there were three of my friends selling cocaine at the party. I decided to get some on credit from one of them – and then another. By

the time midnight rolled around, I had made one lap around the dealers, so as to not work up too large of a bill with any one of them. I
proceeded to do the husbandly thing and called Robin to wish her
"Happy New Year." I informed her that everything was going according to plan. This was the first of many lies that night. I had spent
much more money than I had promised, but I was still planning on being home at 1:00 am. So I engaged my friends on this joyous occasion
and the next thing I knew it was 1:30 am. By this time, I was deep into
my disease and in no way wanted to go home. So I decided to call and
let Robin know that I was playing darts very well, winning lots of
money, and couldn't leave just then. I told her I would be home soon.
She probably knew this was another lie, but she was powerless. This
bought me a couple more hours and, at about 3:30 am, I decided I'd
better give Robin another call. I still did not want to return home so I
told her that I drank too much whiskey and that I really shouldn't be
driving drunk. My addict manipulation had now turned the table so it
was she who wanted me to stay.

At about 5:30 am, with only the other drug addicts and myself left at
the party, I thought I had better get home. The goal now was to get
home before Robin did at about 7:30 am. I called and told her that I
was feeling better and would be home shortly – firmly believing that
this was true. But first, I needed to take a line "for the road." The
next thing I knew, it was 7:30 am, Robin was home, and I was not. I
had done it again. The phone was now ringing often and I knew it was
her because she would be worried. After all, I had told her I was on
my way home two hours earlier. I asked that the host, who was one of
the dealers and the only one beside myself left at the party, not to answer the phone. This was very bad because he was also a friend of my
wife and I was asking him to lie for me by not answering the phone.
He agreed. My addict self-centeredness justified this by asking, "Why
answer the phone now and catch a bunch of anger and grief, and then
have to go through it again when I get home. Just wait and catch it all
when you get home." I later found out Robin called the California
Highway Patrol in desperation wondering if there was a burgundy
240-Z that had gotten in a wreck that night.

I proceeded deeper into the disease. I attempted to create a makeshift
pipe so I could smoke my cocaine; I was on "window patrol" in which I

*obsessively peeked out the window because I was sure there was some-
one outside plotting to get me; I was obsessively crawling on my hands
and knees because I was sure I had dropped a cocaine rock somewhere
(by the way, acoustic ceiling tastes horrible in a crack pipe); and I was
hallucinating to the point I believed there was too much smoke in the
room so we went upstairs and began rifling through a big green gar-
bage bag full of marijuana believing it must be on fire. Looking back on
it, this was nothing short of psychotic behavior.*

*Around 12:00 noon the next day, I finally decided to leave. At this
point, I didn't bother calling Robin because she wouldn't have believed me anyway. I wiped off my sweat and got into the car. I looked
in the rear-view mirror at myself and I had that black-eyed, sunk in,
skeletal look of the "day after." I was sure that if a cop saw me driving in this condition, I would get pulled over. Little did I know that the
cops were actually out there looking for me due to Robin's frightened
phone call to them! As I was driving home, these are the thoughts that
were running through my head: "You idiot! You did it again. You
were only planning on spending $50 and now you are $300 in debt.
All your friends saw just how much of a pitiful addict you are. You
might get pulled over for a DUI and you lied to your wife all night
long. Now, instead of sleeping in and watching the Rose Bowl, you
have to go home and catch a bunch of your wife's anger and sadness
and have to crash because you've been up all night. Happy New Year,
world!" The Big Book describes well the feelings I had that day: "pitiful and incomprehensible demoralization" (Alcoholics Anonymous,
1976, p. 30). I experienced such feelings every time I used. As I tell
you this story, I remember vividly what it felt like and I never, ever,
want to feel like that again. It was horrible.*

Now, had I been thinking about the positive aspects of using and taken
myself through this scenario in thought, I would have switched my focus from the positive aspects of using to the negative ones and would
probably not have entered the craving cycle. As I write this, I can honestly tell you I am very far away from using at this moment. I encourage you to take some time right now to think of a scenario in your life

that you can reflect on when you are locked onto the positive thoughts of using.

Current Dissatisfaction with Sobriety (Awfulizing Sobriety)

The next psychological set-up is *"current dissatisfaction with sobriety."* According to Gorski, "(This) is euphoric recall in reverse... We look at our current sober life and focus upon and exaggerate all of our current pain and discomfort. 'Isn't sobriety awful?' we complain" (Gorski, 1989). Such thoughts arise as: "This sobriety thing isn't all what it's cracked up to be. I don't feel like anything is exciting anymore. All those AA people are a bunch of phonies. I still feel terrible and nothing seems to be improving."

Along with focusing on the negatives of sobriety, "we repress or block out all of the comfort, pleasure and satisfaction that is available to us" (Gorski, 1989). There are many positives you can focus on. Even if you are in very early recovery, the fact you have made a decision to get sober is huge. You deserve to give yourself many positive strokes for that. Do you realize how many like you never make it this far? Many addicts die because their ego and pride prevent them from reaching out for help.

Other positives might be that you're starting to feel better physically. Maybe you are starting to patch up some of your relationships. Maybe you are starting to develop new and positive relationships in your life. Maybe you are starting to gain some hope that you have finally stumbled upon the answer to your problems because you are rubbing elbows with others who have been where you are and now appear to be doing much better. The list goes on. How about the fact that you don't have to experience the physical and emotional hangovers anymore? There is a positive side to every negative. If you can recognize you are being negative about your early sobriety, you can begin to focus on the positives. Many sponsors have their sponsees write a gratitude list in which the addict writes a specified number of things he or she is grateful for. This is a very effective way of creating a positive frame of mind regarding your sobriety. Again, if you can recognize you are focusing on the negatives of recovery, you can simply change your focus to the positives.

At this point, I want to introduce the term *anhedonia* to you. Anhedonia is "the inability to experience pleasure" (Gorski, 1988). This is very common for people in early recovery. My theory is that it results from measuring your current excitement/pleasure level to that which you experienced when you were using. The life of most addicts and alcoholics is exciting. This excitement can result from the rush of the first hit, drink, or pill, the anticipation of it, and the camaraderie that might accompany it. Much of it may be negative excitement like securing your stash, hiding your use, or cleaning up the consequences of it. However, it is excitement all the same. When you get sober, nothing in your sober life comes close to measuring up to that excitement level. A constant feeling of boredom results and you are disillusioned by the fact that you don't have such excitement or pleasure in your life anymore.

The good news is that, as you are removed in time from the memory of the excitement and pleasure levels in your disease, your lower excitement and pleasure levels in early sobriety will be less noticeable in comparison. As a result, it becomes easier for you to get excited and experience pleasure about normal life's events – you are able to again experience excitement and pleasure out of everyday life. The importance of bringing this to your attention is to let you know that if you are experiencing an inability to get excited or experience pleasure in early sobriety, have patience. It is time limited and your excitement and pleasure levels will increase as you are removed in time from the memory of your using days.

When I was only a few days sober and still in a treatment center, my fellow patients and I were taken by hospital van to the alumni Christmas party. I remember being bored out of my mind. I could not believe that any of the alumni could possibly be having as much fun sober as they were exhibiting. I concluded that they must be putting on an act for us newcomers so we would want to stay sober. I wondered whether such an event could ever possibly give me pleasure unless I was loaded.

Approximately eleven months later, I was at my grandmother's house for Thanksgiving. In the past, such gatherings at Grandma's would include my grandfather when he was alive, my father before the divorce, and my uncle before his divorce. They would all play dominoes while some of us kids watched or played with one of Grandpa's gadgets. The moms would all be talking together and my grandmother would typically be playing the piano while bouncing one of us grandchildren on her knee. However, what Thanksgiving had become to me in my using days was getting the meal out of the way so I could get the heck out of there and party uninterrupted for the next four days.

In a very spiritual moment, I started looking around the room. Now my brothers and I were playing dominoes, my grandmother was still playing the piano, and my mom was bouncing my nephew on her knee. I got tears in my eyes and thought, "Isn't this great? It is like old times, but a generation later." For the first time in my sobriety, I realized that I could *get excited about the simple things in life.*

Therefore, it is very important for you to know that the inability to get excited about anything in early sobriety is temporary. As you get removed in time from the memory of the positive and negative excitement of your use, you will once again experience great pleasure and excitement from your life.

> Therefore, it is very important for you to know that the inability to get excited about anything in early sobriety is temporary.

Positive Expectancy

Positive expectancy "is the belief that everything would be fine if we could use drugs again. ...This is a form of 'magical thinking' based upon the mistaken belief that future alcohol and drug use has the power to magically fix our current problems" (Gorski, 1989). This return of denial leads you to think that using will work for you again. "The belief that it will kill us does not destroy the belief that it will work for us again, at least temporarily" (Gorski, 1989). This point was played out for me both professionally and personally:

One day at St. John's Hospital in Santa Monica, I was giving a lecture on the ingredients for recovery and was interrupted by an elderly man who stated, "Bob, I don't have to do all that stuff. My doctor told me that if I have another drink, my liver will fail and I will die – so why would I ever take another drink?" I attempted to explain to him that the decision to stop drinking does not translate directly into not drinking. The decision to stop drinking must translate into the appropriate action, which then leads to not drinking. The group loved this guy and tried to convince him to stay for rehab after detox, but he declined. Three weeks later, we all received the sad news that he drank again and died. Now, it may have been a deterrent if he had believed that one drink would, in fact, cause his liver to fail and he would die. But he probably thought, "Of course one drink will not kill me, so I'll have just one." Of course, we have established the fact that an alcoholic is usually not capable of having just one, so he proceeded to drink himself to death. This is a very important lesson for all of us. People die from the disease of addiction and don't believe it will happen to them. Most of us who work in the addiction profession have witnessed such tragedies more than once.

I also had personal experience with the belief that drugs would kill me, without destroying the belief that they would work for me again. When I used cocaine, I smoked so much that my heart would start hurting severely, and I could not take another hit until it started hurting less. I'm sure I was on the verge of a heart attack, and this happened every time I used. So when I would go through my usual ritual of scoring my drug and cooking it up into the crack cocaine form, I would put the pipe down before I took my first hit and pray to God that it wouldn't kill me this time. Here I was, about to engage in a behavior that I knew could easily take my life, and I was still willing to go through with it. What an insidious disease!

Denial and Evasion

Finally, there is denial and evasion in which "we resist the belief that we are actually doing any of this" (Gorski, 1989). "No, I'm seeing my past use accurately, it really was that good; I'm not awfulizing sobriety, this is really terrible; or, this is not positive expectancy, I'm sure that my using will help me." This is why it is important to have a sober support system that you can share openly with about such distorted thoughts so they can give you a reality check.

Social Set-ups

Social set-up behaviors are easily explained: "We begin to isolate. We avoid social situations and remove ourselves from others. We spend more and more time alone totally preoccupied with self-pity, grandiosity or in black moods" (Gorski, 1989). Many people who come into treatment mistakenly believe that they can attain the necessary recovery information and then get sober on their own. This almost never works. As noted earlier, this is an "I can't," but "we can" program (Gorski, 1989). We must bring others into it and keep them there.

In the last chapter, I referred to what many people in recovery speak of as: "The Committee" in their heads that works against them in their recovery. I believe that this committee is actually the disease itself fighting for its life. This committee tells me what a piece of dirt I am and you are. It is inherently negative, skeptical, and keeps me worrying about and over-reacting to the most trivial events. A sober friend of mine used to share at meetings that the only break he got from his committee was when he went to sleep. Then he would wake up and the first thing his committee would say is, "Where the hell have you been – I've been waiting to talk to you!"

It is important in early sobriety to be very active in working the ingredients for recovery so you can interrupt this committee with reality. However, when you begin to get complacent about your recovery and you begin isolating, this committee is allowed to run uninterrupted. This inevitably leads to relapse. I want to share with you a very common scenario of relapse that many alcoholics and addicts fall into.

Before I got into program management and had my own patient caseload, perhaps my biggest goal for a given client was to get him or her to agree to attend 90 meetings in 90 days. In most cases, I was able to accomplish this. So the person would set out to keep the commitment and attend daily meetings. The person goes to meetings every day for a couple of weeks and then, maybe, doesn't feel well and decides to miss a meeting. So the meeting is missed and daily attendance resumes. The person still feels fine and it does not appear to have had much of an impact on sobriety. However, a message is implanted into the subconscious that reads: "Hmm. I just missed a meeting and still feel okay."

Then another couple of weeks pass and maybe the person wants to attend an event that evening which conflicts with the meeting and decides to miss again. After all, a meeting was missed a few weeks earlier and everything was fine. So the meeting is again missed and the person doesn't feel like going the following night either. The person still feels good despite the fact that the meeting was missed the day before so decides to miss again. Now two straight meetings have been missed and the person still feels fine. Meeting attendance resumes and, again, a message is planted in the subconscious that reads: "Hmm. I missed two meetings in a row and I still feel okay." Do you see where this is going? These missed meetings increase in frequency and the person still feels fine. In fact, the person might eventually miss meetings for a week straight and still feel okay. The person begins to think: "Hmm. I've missed meetings for a week straight and I still feel great." The person then thinks that maybe going to so many meetings is necessary for some people, but it does not seem necessary for him/her. The person might decide that one meeting weekly is adequate and begins doing just that. However, the progression continues and, eventually, the person doesn't feel like attending the weekly meeting and decides not to. Now the person has not gone to a meeting for two weeks. Members of his or her support system begin to call wondering why the person is not showing up at meetings. But the addict screens his or her calls to avoid the embarrassment of not working a program because deep down feels he/she should be attending more meetings. So the person is not going to meetings, not having any contact with his or her sober support system and "the committee" has been allowed to run uninterrupted for an extended period of time. The addict thinking and behavior ensues and, the next thing the addict knows, he or she has relapsed and wonders how this happened. I see this scenario happen very often.

I might add here that going to meetings is like putting recovery in the bank. Attending on a daily basis gives you plenty of recovery to draw upon in difficult times. When you first stop going to meetings, it is as if you are withdrawing recovery from your account without depositing any. As long as you still have recovery to draw upon, you often continue to feel all right. However, if you continue to make withdrawals without any deposits, you eventually have nothing left to draw upon and you relapse.

Trigger Events

Terence Gorski defines a trigger event as "any internal or external occurrence that activates a craving (obsession, compulsion, physical
craving, and drug-seeking behavior)" (Gorski, 1988). In breaking
down this definition, "internal" occurrences are thoughts or feelings,
and "external" occurrences involve the five senses: sight, sound, smell,
taste, and touch. In order for it to be a trigger, such an event must be
connected in some way to your using. The event must also happen just
before, or simultaneous to, the actual use (Gorski, 1988).

A simple way of explaining this is by relating it to classical (or Pavlovian) conditioning. Ivan Pavlov was a Russian scientist who won the
Nobel Peace Prize in 1904 for his research in digestive processes.
While studying the relationship between salivation and digestive processes in dogs, he would show the dog some meat powder causing it to
salivate and then measured the salivation level. One day, Dr. Pavlov
noticed that the dogs were starting to salivate as soon as he entered the
room. It appeared that there was some relationship created between
him and the meat powder. To study this phenomenon, he rang a bell
just prior to showing the dog the meat powder and would again measure the salivation level. He did this repeatedly: bell → meat powder
→ salivation, bell → meat powder → salivation, etc. He eventually
found that he could ring the bell, not present the meat powder, and the
dog would still salivate. Thus, there was a connection made for the
dog between the bell and the meat powder that prompted the salivation
(PageWise, 2002). For our purposes, the bell was the event (trigger)
that occurred just before, or simultaneous to, the presentation of the
meat powder, which caused the dog to salivate, or crave, the meat
powder. The challenge for you is to identify the bells (triggers) that
cause you to salivate (crave) your drug of choice. This will allow you
to avoid or manage such triggers. We will now explore, in more de-
tail, the different types of triggers that Gorski identifies as being
strongly associated with craving.

Thinking Triggers

Thinking about using becomes a trigger when it is repeatedly followed by actual use. I don't know about you, but when I thought about using, I used. I never thought about using and said to myself, "That doesn't sound like a very good idea, I don't think I'll do that." Therefore, whenever I thought about using, I did. So there was a connection made between my thinking about using and my using. Thus, thinking about using was a trigger.

Gorski warns against repressing such thoughts when they arise because they simply get stored away and come back stronger later (Gorski, 1988). This usually happens when you are in a weak emotional place. After all, if you repress such thoughts, aren't you really doing the same thing you were doing when you were out there using? You had an uncomfortable thought or feeling and you shoved it down with drugs or alcohol so you could pretend it wasn't there. However, such repression is very common because, when you begin thinking of using, your first instinct is to avoid the thought because you are in recovery and don't want to relapse.

Gorski suggests processing thoughts of using in a controlled setting with a counselor (1988). Processing can also be done by calling your sponsor (or another member of your sober support system) and talking about it. This way, together, you can make some sense out of the using thought and, if done correctly, you will come to the conclusion that using is not such a good idea after all. Consequently, the using thought goes away because it then lacks merit.

I have a rather unorthodox way of illustrating this point. Imagine a big drum sitting next to you that is jam-packed with 50 thoughts of using. These thoughts are so tightly packed inside the drum it is ready to burst. You might look at the drum bursting as signifying relapse. Since this drum is so tightly packed, these thoughts of using leak out of the drum, one by one, and enter your head. When thought number one leaks out, there is a decision to be made. You can either process the thought by using the program tools as mentioned previously, or you can shove the thought right back into the drum and close the lid. If you decide on the latter, you still have 50 thoughts left in the drum and it is still jam-packed. However, if you opt to process this thought and make some sense of it, you get to dispose of it and now you have only 49 thoughts of using left in the drum. When the next thought leaks out, you have a similar decision to make. If you decide to keep processing such thoughts, the drum will begin emptying out. Let's say that you have adequately processed 20 such thoughts and there are only 30 remaining. Now the drum is not jam-packed and the thoughts don't leak out as often. Additionally, when the next thought does leak out, you are not thrown into so much of a panic because you know that you have successfully dealt with such thoughts on several previous occasions. Your reaction then might sound something like this, "Okay, here's another one of these pesky thoughts of using. I'll simply do what I usually do and call my sponsor." Your conversation with your sponsor might sound something like this, "Hi, George. I am having another one of my thoughts of using. No big deal. I don't really feel like using and these are the reasons why I shouldn't...." So the thoughts come less frequently and they don't have nearly the impact on you as they used to. What eventually happens is a process called extinction. Your thoughts of using now become associated with your not using, rather than your using, and such thoughts no longer trigger you. Going back to Pavlovian theory, it would be like: ring the bell → no meat powder; ring the bell → no meat powder. Pretty soon the dog is going to think, "Yeah right, this bell doesn't mean anything." The connection has been broken.

Feeling Triggers

A feeling trigger is "any emotional state that was linked with the drug use" (Gorski, 1988). Any feeling that is repeatedly followed by using drugs or alcohol becomes a feeling trigger. A common feeling trigger is anger. If, whenever you felt angry you drank whiskey, there was a connection made between your anger and whiskey. So whenever you get angry in sobriety, it triggers you to want to drink whiskey. Another example is the feeling of shame. If your feelings of shame or embarrassment led to your taking pills, a connection is made between shame and taking pills. Thus, shame would become a trigger for taking pills. The feeling doesn't necessarily need to be a negative feeling. In fact, some of my biggest triggers were positive feelings, such as my propensity to use cocaine when I got excited, or to use marijuana when I felt accomplished or deserving of a reward. I'll never forget the first time I mowed the lawn in sobriety. My craving for marijuana was overwhelming.

Acting or Behavioral Triggers

Acting triggers are things that you *do* that are connected to your using, such as: going to bars, visiting using people, or going to your favorite liquor store (Gorski, 1988.) You have some control over these triggers because they result from your behavior. Therefore, you can and should avoid these triggers right away. As mentioned earlier, a drug addict or alcoholic has absolutely no business getting into a drinking or using situation. You need to avoid them at all cost. This is especially true in early sobriety. Eventually, you will be able to handle some such situations, but that will happen later in sobriety and we will explore this later in the chapter.

Relating or Interactional Triggers

Relating or interactional triggers can involve certain relationships (Gorski, 1988.) We can use the stereotypical example: Whenever you were around your in-laws, you needed to have a drink. So visiting your in-laws would then become a trigger for drinking. Another relating trigger is using drugs other than your drug of choice (Gorski, 1988). For example, if whenever you drank alcohol you used cocaine, alcohol would become a trigger for cocaine use. What could be a bigger trigger for a mind-altering substance than another mind-altering substance?

A little over two years before I got sober, I took a trip to Lake Nacamiento to go water-skiing over the Fourth of July weekend. I was very much looking forward to water-skiing with my wife and friends. However, I was so deep into my disease, I never once made it to the water. We binged on cocaine literally the whole four days we were there. Interestingly, the brother of a very close friend of ours who used to keep right up with us in the partying category didn't hang out with us and went water-skiing all weekend. I was very intrigued (and jealous) about this, so I approached him and asked what had happened. He explained that he had been through rehab and how the 12-Step pro-

grams had helped him. It all sounded doable to me except when he got to the part that I would have to quit drinking and smoking pot if I expected to stay off of cocaine. My response, as I remember it, was something like this, "Wait a minute, I just have a little cocaine problem. I don't need to take it to that extreme." Well, it took me two more years of painful research in my disease to become willing to go to that extreme. I now know that he was absolutely right and he eventually became my sponsor when I got sober. I have not seen one person come into treatment and have success at stopping one drug while continuing to use the others for any extended period of time without eventually returning to his or her drug of choice.

Dreams of drinking or using are also triggers of significance. These dreams are common in early recovery, seem very realistic, and can be scary. I will distinguish between two types of using dreams. The first, and most dangerous to the recovering addict, is the dream in which you are getting ready to drink or use and suddenly wake up. My experience is that there is often an extreme level of disappointment when you wake up and realize that you can't use. These dreams are so real that you actually experience the physical and emotional feelings you felt just before using. There may be no stronger trigger than waking up with these feelings. This is an extremely dangerous place to be. It is very important, especially in your early recovery, to have someone in your sober support system whom you can call at any time day or night. When waking up from such a dream, I highly recommend you call such a person immediately so you can talk your way through the trigger.

The other type of dream is one in which you find yourself having already relapsed. Again, the dreams are so real that you experience all the emotions you would if a relapse actually occurred, including sadness, shame, and remorse. Very often the thoughts that are running through your head in such a dream include rationalization and minimization, i.e. "That wasn't a relapse because it wasn't my drug of choice." Other thoughts often include wondering if you are going to be honest about the relapse and evaluating what the consequences of the relapse will be. When you awaken from the dream, you are typically very relieved that it was only a dream. I remember rejoicing in such a situation. This type of dream can be very therapeutic because you actually experience the uncomfortable feelings associated with re-lapse, without actually relapsing.

I can remember only one time where I was actually using in my dream. The whole dream was the preparation for a hit of crack cocaine. In the dream, I finally took the hit. As I reached my maximum lung ca-pacity, I suddenly woke up. This dream was so real that I woke up with my lungs completely full of air and actually holding my breath. I remember looking at Robin sleeping next to me and turning my head quickly away from her and exhaling! I even had a small placebo effect as I actually got a little rush when I exhaled!

Finally, I want to share with you one final item in regards to using dreams. There was a time in my early recovery that I was having such dreams every night. I was getting very tired of this and shared at eve-ry meeting about them. One day a guy approached me after a meeting who stated that he had the same problem in his early recovery. He stated that during one such dream he was offered cocaine and actually turned it down. He very rarely had using dreams after that one. He shared this with me hoping that I might have the same experience. I did!

Recovering from Triggers

According to Gorski, there are three phases in the trigger recovery pro-cess. Phase I is to "eliminate as many of them as you can, for a limited period of time, until (you are) stable" (Gorski, 1988). Again, in very early sobriety, you do not go to bars or other using places, you avoid people who use and drink, and you avoid any other triggers you may be aware of. A list of common triggers can be found at the end of this chapter.

"The second phase is a gradual reintroduction of the triggers so that the person can learn how to cope with them" (Gorski, 1988). This does not mean to gradually re-introduce you into the crack house or your favorite watering hole, but there are some trigger situations that you should be able to eventually participate in. As stated earlier, alco-hol permeates our society and you would have to live a very sheltered life in order to avoid it over the long term. Therefore, in order to lead any kind of a normal life, gradual re-introduction to some trigger situations is necessary. This re-introduction process is best done with your sponsor's involvement or with your therapist or group if you have one. Following is an example of this process in my sobriety.

When I was about 90 days sober and still involved in the aftercare portion of my treatment program, we were invited to the wedding of my wife's cousin in Chandler, Arizona. I thought I'd really like to go. However, I had learned from past experience that decisions I made on my own in relation to my sobriety were typically bad ones. So I decided to leave it completely up to my group. So I attended my next group session and put it out to them. The consensus was that since I was still working a very strong sobriety program, going to daily meetings, and going with my supportive wife, I could probably stay sober if I created a sobriety plan. The group then proceeded to help me put this plan together.

First, they suggested that I carry a Big Book onto the plane. The thinking was that since flying on an airplane was a trigger for me to drink, it would be difficult to order a drink while holding a Big Book in my hand. The book has an embossed cover so nobody would know what it was and, if they recognized it, they probably have one and I might meet someone in the program.

The next suggestion was to go to 12-Step meetings each day I was in Arizona. They had me call the downtown Los Angeles Central Office of AA to get the number of the central office in Chandler, Arizona. I was to get a meeting scheduled for each day I was there and, if possible, schedule a meeting for the time of the reception so if I got into trouble, I could simply leave the reception and go to a meeting. In fact, this actually happened:

At the reception, I found myself talking to my wife's uncle next to the wet bar at his home. All of a sudden, someone plopped down a bottle of my favorite whiskey onto the bar right in front of me. After recovering from my slight panic, I excused myself and informed my wife that I was going to a meeting. Fortunately, and I suggest this highly, I got the address and directions from the AA Central Office which made it easy for me to go.

I went to the meeting and took a 90-day chip in celebration of my sobriety time. As opposed to meetings in California where a key chain or a coin is usually given in acknowledgment of various lengths of sobriety, their chip was actually a marble. I asked them if there was any significance to using a marble. I was told to carry it with me all the time and if I get the urge to drink, take it out of my pocket and throw it as far as I can. The thinking was that by the time I found it, I might not want to drink anymore. I asked someone else and I was told that if I want to drink, go ahead and pour the drink and put the marble into it. When it dissolves, I can drink it. So much for Arizona humor!

After the meeting I ended up going back to the reception where everyone was having a great time dancing. This really looked fun to me but I had never danced sober before. I always had to have at least a few drinks in me before I could dance because I was not a very good dancer and cared too much about what other people thought of me. When I had a few drinks, I felt like I danced like John Travolta and I didn't give a damn what anyone thought. So I concocted a plan to wait for a fast song that I liked, run and slide onto the dance floor while playing "air guitar" and, hopefully, begin dancing. So a Van Halen song came on and I was off and running. Little did I know that just after I left for my meeting, the bride and groom arrived, walked across the portable dance floor, and everyone followed tradition by throwing rice at them. You can imagine what happened next. As I attempted to slide onto the dance floor, my feet hit the rice and came right out from under me. I hit the floor, followed by two of my wife's female cousins (one of them the bride!) who I managed to take down with me – one of them right onto my lap. As I rose to my feet, my face must have been beet red and, as I looked around the dance floor, I could see my wife's family's reaction which I perceived as, "There he goes, he's drunk again" – and I was probably the only sober person there!

Anyway, other elements of my sobriety plan consisted of calling my sponsor each day I was there and reading the Big Book for a half-hour each evening. Upon returning, my group and I processed what worked, and what additional program tools I might have used, so I could use them the next time I might have to expose myself to triggers.

Through such a process, I was able to participate in increasingly more activities in my sobriety to the point that I can now do almost anything without being triggered. This is due to the third phase of the trigger recovery process called the "extinguishing process" (Gorski, 1988). As mentioned earlier, triggers become extinguished when repeated exposure to them is connected with not drinking, rather than drinking. As noted above, in relating it to Pavlovian theory, it would be like: ring the bell → no meat powder; ring the bell → no meat powder, etc. Eventually the dog comes to learn that the bell doesn't mean anything and it is not affected by it anymore.

Following is a list of common triggers that I have compiled over the years during my trigger lectures at treatment centers I have worked at. During such lectures, I stand at the blackboard writing down what patients see as their triggers. In each lecture, we come up with about 30 to 40 triggers that are written on the board. A member of the group writes these triggers down on paper and it is photocopied and distributed. The group members are then asked to highlight which triggers they think especially apply to them. It is recommended to them to review this list of triggers on a daily basis. I encourage you to do the same with this list:

Triggers List

Shame
Fear
Cash
People that drink or use
Drinking or using places
Social engagements
Anxiety
Sporting events
Sex
Family
Depression
Boredom
Accomplishment
Anger/resentments
Financial problems
Comfort
Laziness
Isolation
Loneliness
Negativity
Movies
Smells
Seeing drugs or alcohol
Excitement
Books/magazines
School
Idle time
Rejection
Meals
Refrigerator
Using or drinking lingo

Paraphernalia
Work
Time of day, week, month, year
Holidays
Vacations
Grief/loss
Change
Birthdays
Music
Self-pity
Using memories/fantasizing
Fatigue
Glamorizing use
Mouthwash
Advertisements
Old behavior
Using dreams
Telephone
Drinking/using "war stories"
Games
Using rituals
Purchasing places
Caffeine
Work quitting time
Commercials
Clothes
Hobbies
Marital problems
Dieting
Pawnable items
Certain foods

Hunger/thirst
Neighborhoods
Pornography
Taste
Happiness
Chemical withdrawal
Weather
Dishonesty
Police
Payday
Gambling
Other addictions
Flying
Travel
Concerts
Illness
Physical pain
Violence
Pagers
Seeing others loaded
Insomnia
Anniversaries
Smoke
Sounds
Billboards
Driving
Failure
Doctor's office
Television
ATMs
Spiritual emptiness

Warning Signs

Terence Gorski also coined the term "warning signs". In his book, *Staying Sober*, he writes that he conducted clinical interviews with 118 recovering alcoholics and drug addicts who had completed a 21 or 28-day program, recognized they were addicted, intended on staying sober post-discharge with the help of AA and outpatient counseling, and eventually relapsed. By compiling the responses of these subjects identifying the warning signs that might have told them they were on the road to relapse, he came up with a list of the most common responses – hence, the creation of Gorski's famous 37 Warning Signs of Relapse (Gorski and Miller, 1986, p.140).

The importance of warning sign identification is based on the idea that relapse is not the *event* of picking up drugs or alcohol. Relapse is a *process* that happens over days, weeks, months, or even years and finally culminates in the actual use. This is good news for people in recovery because the intention is to avoid the "picking up" part. Warning signs can tell you that you are in the relapse process. If you can identify such warning signs when they occur, you can intervene on them before you actually pick up.

It is important to identify your warning signs early in recovery because when you are in the relapse process, you have a tendency to have distorted thinking which makes identification of relapse warning signs extremely difficult. If you regularly view a list of warning signs you compiled when you were not in the relapse process, you will be able to identify symptoms you might not otherwise be capable of recognizing.

Warning signs and triggers are not the same, although there is much overlap between them. Remember, a trigger is something that is connected to your using and activates the craving cycle. A warning sign is something that indicates that you may be on the road to relapse. For example, seeing using friends can be both a trigger and a warning sign. As a trigger, seeing using friends often occurs simultaneous to, or just before, using drugs or alcohol. A connection is made between seeing using friends, and drinking or using. This connection is what activates the craving cycle and makes it a trigger. Seeing using friends may also be a warning sign of relapse because exposing yourself to such people is dangerous to your sobriety. Exposing yourself to such danger is clearly a warning sign that you are setting yourself up for relapse.

Following is a list of warning signs that I compiled in a similar fashion to my compilation of triggers. In my relapse prevention education series, clients are asked to identify warning signs that might have indicated they were on the road to relapse. If they had no relapse history, they are asked to identify what warning signs they think might occur for them prior to relapse. If you purchase Gorski's *Staying Sober,* you will notice much overlap in these and his original 37 Warning Signs.

Warning Signs

Isolating
Decrease in meetings
Quick temper
Justifying
Fantasizing
Ignorance
Decrease in life structure
Minimizing
Over-sleeping
Obsession
Old behavior
Increased anxiety
Overconfidence
Decreased exercise
Apathy
Breaking commitments
Decreased phone calls
Dishonesty
Insomnia
Increased selfishness
Major changes
Increased fear
Visiting purchasing places
Sloth
Projecting
Sense of entitlement
Impatience

Loneliness
Not listening
Other compulsions
Mood-swings
Hanging with users
Return of denial
Procrastination
Poor diet
Hanging in using places
Increased self-will
Planning use
Increased fatigue
Complacency
Decreased step work
Negative thinking
Defensiveness
Decreased willingness
Hoarding money
Increased irritability
Taking other's inventory
Hopelessness
Increased confusion
Stubbornness
Arrogance
Self-pity
Sobriety loses priority

Decreased sponsor contact
Increased anger/resentment
Rationalizing
Seeking negative excitement
Increase in ego
Decreased spiritual program
Decreased hygiene
Stopping psych medication
Refusing help
Increased craving
Increased depression
Lack of sleep
Increased boredom
Feeling overwhelmed
Comparing self to others
Increased guilt/shame
Increased sadness
Shutting people out
Not open about feelings
Lack of gratitude
Early recovery "relationships"
Desperation
Drinking non-alcoholic beer
Decreased 12 step reading
Decrease in hobby activity
Decreased journal writing

As with the relapse triggers, I encourage you to either photocopy this list or copy it down on a sheet of paper. Then highlight which warning signs might particularly apply to you. In addition to this, make a copy of the ingredients for recovery at the end of chapter two. You will then have a copy of the ingredients for recovery, relapse triggers, and relapse warning signs. I want to encourage you, as I do my patients, to keep these lists accessible so you can view them on a daily basis. I recommend putting them with your morning meditation book and starting your day with the morning meditation reading and then reviewing these lists. This review will not take more than five minutes a day and it is an invaluable resource for your recovery.

CHAPTER 6
THE 12 STEPS

*P*rior to my inpatient treatment stay, I had been to a couple of 12-Step meetings and some addicts spoke of the 12 Steps and sponsorship, but I had not been to enough meetings to fully understand what they were all about and what might be accomplished by working them. While in treatment, I worked the first three steps and heard counselors and alumni referring to them, but nobody really took me through each step so I could really understand how they work. When I was approximately 90 days sober, I went to a Cocaine Anonymous speaker meeting. The speaker had about five years sobriety, which at the time seemed like forever to me. In the midst of his sharing, he began describing his journey through the 12 Steps. While this speaker shared his experience with each of them, and how they helped him in his recovery, I was glued to my seat. When he was finished, I felt I finally knew what the steps were about and how they would help me not only stay sober, but to gain some serenity in my life.

I must tell you I had a lot of fear about working the steps. It was not so much the work involved, but I feared that I would work them and still feel the emptiness I felt my entire life. It was as if by not working them, I would still have an ace in the hole in case things got bad enough. If I worked the steps and they didn't work, I would no longer have hope. The pitch by the above speaker gave me the courage to proceed. It is my hope that the following review of the steps might do the same for you.

I need to preface this by letting you know that I am not speaking as an expert on AA or the steps, but through my personal and professional experience, I have gained much insight into their workings. Most of what I am about to share with you I have learned from people with many years of sobriety and from my own experience with working them. The 12 Steps can be found in their entirety in the Big Book (Alcoholics Anonymous, 2001, pp. 59-60).

Step 1: We admitted we were powerless over alcohol – that our lives had become unmanageable.

This step is placed first for a very important reason. If you thought you had the power to get sober on your own, why would you need anyone's help? Additionally, if you have not come to the conclusion that your life has been negatively affected by your using, why would you have a need to stop? As you might gather from these statements, this step is divided into two parts.

The first part is admitting to yourself that you are powerless over alcohol (or your drug of choice). This admission includes your powerlessness over that first drink, and over what happens afterward. Many in the program state that it is the first drink that gets you drunk. This is true because most alcoholics cannot stop at just one, so they inevitably get drunk once they take that first drink.

Admitting you're powerlessness over alcohol (or drugs) is essential if you are to stay sober. You need to believe this to the core of your very being. If you have any doubt about your inability to control your use, you will surely try it again. This disease is so strong, it will latch onto the slightest doubt you have and convince you that you can drink or use without the usual consequences. Regarding the desire to drink like normal people, the Big Book reads: "The persistence of this illusion is astonishing" (Alcoholics Anonymous, 2001, p. 30).

This statement reflects my own experience. I have proved my powerlessness hundreds of times. However, every time I made the decision to use, I thought I would be able to control it. Once I crossed the line into addiction, I never, ever, succeeded at doing this. As we will see later, Step 2 alludes to the insane nature of our disease. I learned the following definition of insanity in the program: "Trying the same thing over and over again and expecting different results." After repeated failures at trying to drink or use like normal people, we try it again. How insane is this type of behavior? Amazing!

The second part of Step 1 is admitting your life has become unmanageable. This is important for at least two reasons. First, as mentioned earlier, if you don't see your life as being negatively affected by your use, a change will not seem necessary. Second, the extent of change necessary to achieve sobriety will not be achieved without the desperation resulting from fear of further consequences of your use.

In the midst of your disease, it is often difficult to see all the consequences of your use. This is partly due to the fact that you are not thinking straight in your addiction. It is also due to your disease, or "committee," constantly keeping your focus on whatever part of your life that appears to be at least somewhat manageable, for example: holding down a job or marriage. It is only when you get the substance out of your system, and honestly work Step 1, that you can truly see your life for what it is – a mess.

A strategy that I often use in treatment with clients who exhibit such denial is to have them present their drug/alcohol history and consequences assignment up at the chalkboard for everyone to see. They write such consequences on the board and the group aids them in identifying additional consequences they may have forgotten. This was particularly effective for one elderly gentleman who deemed himself a "functional alcoholic." Once the list was complete, the group was asked to sit in silence and observe what became a very extensive list. The man was then asked, "Do these look like the consequences of a functional alcoholic?" The truth was undeniable. He admitted at that point that his life was, in fact, unmanageable. This was a huge breakthrough for him and it cleared the way for a desire to change. Such an exercise, in some form, is usually done with your sponsor as you work Step 1.

Once you have made the above admissions in Step 1, you are left with a dilemma. If you have admitted your powerlessness and unmanageability, you are admitting that you cannot do it alone. This clears the way for Step 2.

Step 2: Came to believe that a Power greater than ourselves could restore us to sanity.

There are two parts to this step also. Not only do you need to believe in a Higher Power, but you must also come to believe that this Power is able to relieve you of your addiction.

This step comes very easy for some people. Many have believed in such a Power all of their lives. However, this step drives fear into some people and repulses others. Some people have never believed in such a Power and being asked to suddenly believe in one is no small request. Others may have grown up with religious beliefs but were so turned off by the hypocrisy that is often present, they decided they want no part of it.

The good news here is that the "Power" can be one of your own under-standing. You do not have to subscribe to the ideas of any particular religion, nor the to ideas of anyone else. You come to believe in a Higher Power that works for *you*. This leaves the possibilities wide open. The important thing here is to have an open mind to the idea. If you will allow yourself to have an open mind, you will come to believe in something that can work. Later in this chapter you will find examples of Higher Powers that others have used which might help you find one. Keep in mind that many of your own ideas have not worked in attaining sobriety. Since you have not yet been successful, you may want to start following the direction of others who have been success-ful at it. As I mentioned earlier, these are mainstream ideas that millions have used to attain their own sobriety.

Start by remembering your plight. When you work Step 1, you admit that you cannot quit using on your own. You have likely put yourself, and others, through an enormous amount of pain through your addiction. Doesn't the thought of getting your life back appear attractive by now? Wouldn't you do just about anything to stop the pain? You have probably done more outlandish things in your using than surrendering some of your old ideas to clear the way to get your life back. Isn't it worth a try? What have you got to lose?

Many people are able to get over this hurdle by observing those maintaining sobriety who have turned to a Higher Power for help. If you take an honest look at such people, it will become very apparent that they have more peace than you are experiencing. You might ask yourself at that point, "Wouldn't it be nice to have that kind of serenity?" If you attend meetings regularly, you will find hundreds of people who have taken this course of action and have achieved sobriety. You will also hear stories of how they broke the barrier you may now struggle with. If you are honest with yourself, it will be easy to see the sense in taking a similar path instead of continuing to be unwilling to take this step. Don't take the path of others who refuse to be willing and need to go out and create more consequences through their continued use before obtaining such willingness.

I would like to clarify here that AA, and the other 12-Step programs are not religious programs – they are spiritual programs. As mentioned earlier, religious organizations believe in a certain God and, typically, have specified ritualistic practices. On the contrary, people who are working the 12-Step programs have their own idea of a Higher Power and the way they choose to interact with their Higher Power is a personal choice. As noted earlier, some in the program make a distinction that religion is man-made, and spirituality is God-made. In 12-Step recovery, you may see that spirituality is simply the presence of God and the result of His presence.

In this light, you may come to see that spirituality is simply an awareness of the presence of a Higher Power. When you are feeling spiritual, God is in the room with you. You may believe that God is always there, but you are not always aware of His presence. During times when you are aware of His presence, you typically think and act the way you believe God wants you to think and act. Additionally, this awareness will bring you much peace because you know God is in control and taking care of you. During times when you are not aware of God's presence, you typically feel very fearful and vulnerable. This fear is dangerous to addicts like us because we often anesthetize it through our drug and alcohol use.

Chapter 4 in the "Big Book" entitled, "We Agnostics" is also very helpful for many who struggle with this step. Toward the end of the chapter, an alcoholic struggling with the Higher Power issue finally started considering the possibility of a Higher Power by asking himself the question, "Is it possible that all the religious people I have known are wrong?" Finally the thought hit him, "Who are you to say there is no God?" (Alcoholics Anonymous, 2001, p. 56). Therefore, being a mere speck of humanity in this huge universe, you might begin to ask yourself how you can be so sure there is no Higher Power? So, if you cannot be sure one way or the other, why not open up your mind to an idea that might save your life?

If you are struggling with this step, I hope you have come to the point in your life where you have made a decision to at least be open-minded about it. This willingness alone will open the door for a new way of life for you. Here are some examples of what some alcoholics and addicts have used for their Higher Power:

- The Higher Power associated with one's religion
- The power of AA as a whole (meetings)
- The power of nature
- The power of good
- A mountain
- The ocean
- Higher Power not otherwise specified
- The Power of cause and effect

Remember, if you can simply get yourself to become *willing* to identify a Higher Power, you will find one. The only times people fail at identifying one is if they fail at achieving such willingness. So open up your mind and work on getting your life back!

Step 3: Made a decision to turn our will and our lives over to the care of God *as we understood Him.*

When you come to the conclusion that there is a Higher Power that can defeat your disease, you are ready for the all-important Step 3. To turn your will and your life over to God is to give up what *you* want for what God wants. Alcoholics and addicts in the

> To turn your will and your life over to God is to give up what *you* want for what God wants.

throes of their illness have a tendency to be very controlling, selfish, and self-centered. As a result, turning over our needs for what God wants is a very difficult task. In fact, this task is virtually impossible for most of us. We are just not capable of doing that for any extended period of time. Additionally, if you were truly able to accomplish this, you would not need meetings, a sponsor, the rest of the steps, or any of the other program tools because you would be a "spiritual giant" who had no need for them.

Therefore, the most important part of this step is the first three words: "Made a decision." To complete this step, all you have to do is make a decision to turn your will and life over to a Higher Power. This makes Step 3 much more reasonable than many people make it out to be. Once you have made this decision, Steps 4-9 are then worked to re-move whatever gets in the way of your accomplishing what you "made a decision" to do in Step 3.

Step 3 is the centerpiece around which all of the steps revolve. You work Steps 1 and 2 to prepare yourself for Step 3, and you work the rest of the steps to accomplish what you made a decision to do in Step 3. If you turn your will and life over to a Higher Power, you attain a serenity level that allows you to stay off alcohol and drugs. You final-ly live a life feeling comfortable in your own skin. As mentioned ear-lier, this is a process, not a destination. As you continue to practice the principles of this program, you will be able to turn your will and life over to your Higher Power for increasingly longer periods of time.

How this plays out in my own life is as follows. After I get up and take a shower in the morning, I sit on my bed and read the before-mentioned morning meditation passage for that day. I then spend some time thanking God for my sobriety and asking Him for still an-other day of abstinence. I then proceed to do my best at giving up my will for God's will through prayer. It might sound something like this, "Dear God, please allow me to give up my needs for what you want today. Please show me what your will is so that it can be done through me. I have screwed things up so bad in the past, Lord, that I really need you to continue to take over. Please help me to recognize when I am taking control back so I can return it to you. Oh dear God, please take care of me today and allow me the strength to do your will." When I do this, a calm feeling comes over me. My serenity level in starting my day is in direct proportion to my sincerity in saying this prayer.

Turning your will and life over to God's care does not relieve you of life's responsibilities – you still have to do the footwork according to what you believe God wants you to do that day. However, it does relieve you of the responsibility for the results. You need to take what you believe to be appropriate action in your life and leave the results business up to God. This way of living provides tremendous relief. Most of us worry so much about so many things. Giving God the responsibility for what happens in His world gives you indescribable peace. This should be great news for you. All you will be responsible for is the footwork and you no longer have to worry about the results because God is going to take care of it.

To aid in the process of understanding Step 3, read from the personal story by Dr. Paul entitled: *Acceptance Was the Answer* on page 417 (or page 449 in the 3rd edition) of the "Big Book." In his story, Dr. Paul describes how acceptance of his alcoholism was the key to his recovery. He then goes on to say:

> "And acceptance is the answer to *all* my problems today. When I am disturbed, it is because I find some person, place, thing, or situation – some fact of my life –unacceptable to me, and I can find no serenity until I accept that person, place, thing or situation as being exactly the way it is supposed to be at this moment. Nothing, absolutely nothing, happens in God's world by mistake. Until I could accept my alcoholism, I could not stay sober; unless I accept life completely on life's terms, I cannot be happy. I need to concentrate not so much on what needs to be changed in the world as on what needs to be changed in me and my attitudes.

> Shakespeare said, 'All the world's a stage, all the men and women merely players.' He forgot to mention that I was the chief critic. I was always able to see the flaw in every person, every situation. And I was always glad to point it out, because I knew you wanted perfection, just as I did. AA and acceptance

have taught me that there is a bit of good in the worst of us and a bit of bad in the best of us; that we are all children of God and we each have a right to be here. When I complain about me or about you, I am complaining about God's handiwork. I am saying that I know better than God (Alcoholics Anonymous, 2001, p. 417)."

That last sentence floored me when I first read it. To me this means that, if I do not like something that is happening in this world, I am telling God He doesn't know what He's doing! When I am able to live by this page on acceptance, I am able to effectively cope with anything that comes my way. As you can see, the above passage on acceptance very much relates to what we are trying to accomplish in making our decision in Step 3. Acceptance is the key if I am going to be able to give up my will for God's.

When you are tested in some way by the happenings in God's world, you might ask yourself, "Hmm. I wonder why God has placed this situation in my life?" or "I wonder what God has in mind here?" You might be able to find some very positive reasons why God allows certain events in other's lives and your own. In fact, you might even find some enjoyment out of trying to figure it out. Sometimes you might simply chalk it up to God's sense of humor. However, when tragic things happen in this world, it is very difficult to come up with a good reason why God might be allowing it. This is especially true when someone suffers or dies a premature death (by the way, toward the end of my writing the original draft of this book, the World Trade Center and the Pentagon were attacked). What might help during such times is considering the possibility that, being human, you are only aware of the human realm of reality. Since you are not God, you do not know everything. And if you believe God is good, it follows that you would agree He must be able to see something that you cannot. Maybe when you die, you will move to a realm with a broader scope and be able to understand what is really happening when such tragedy presents itself. Maybe pain and suffering is very minute in the big picture. My intention here is not to present such ideas as truths, but to share with you the infinite possibilities that appear once you begin living a spiritual life.

Finally, I'd like to share with you a short version of the first three steps which simplifies them:

> Step 1) I can't
> Step 2) He can
> Step 3) Let Him

Step 4: Made a searching and fearless moral inventory of ourselves.

Once you have made the necessary "decision" in Step 3, you are ready to get down to the real work with the help of a Higher Power's guidance. This work will remove what gets in the way of your accomplishing what you have decided to do in Step 3. As the words "searching" and "fearless" imply, you need to be brave enough to look past your emotional defenses and be honest with yourself about who you are and how you operate. This is a difficult task for most of us because we have been lying to ourselves for years. If we were to be honest with ourselves about our shortcomings, we would then have to deal with the associated feelings. Instead, we often use chemicals to distort our perceptions of ourselves and to numb our feelings. One of the keys to recovery is getting honest with ourselves and utilizing the tools of recovery to tolerate such feelings. Therefore, while we learn to get honest with ourselves and deal with the associated feelings, we no longer have a reason to run to chemicals. Through this process, we learn we can tolerate feelings through the support of our peers and can deal with the feelings as they come, rather than building up a whole new inventory of lies to ourselves. Remember to employ Step 3 in this process. Ask for willingness, open-mindedness, honesty, and guidance to discover the truth about yourself.

On page 64 of the *Alcoholics Anonymous* (2001), it reads that, in order for a business to be successful, it must face the facts regarding the stock in trade. In the same way, in order for us to be successful, we need to face the facts about ourselves – positive and negative. It also speaks of the "self, manifested in various ways, was what

> "Resentment is the 'number one' offender.
> It destroys more alcoholics than anything else."

had defeated us" and that we need to look at what forms this takes. "Resentment is the 'number one' offender. It destroys more alcoholics than anything else. From it stems all forms of spiritual disease, for we have been not only mentally and physically ill, we have been spiritually sick." The Big Book suggests that we write a list of "people, institutions, or principles" that we are resentful toward, the cause of these resentments, and why we are resentful toward them. On page 65 is an example of how this can be done on a sheet of paper using three columns. Regarding why we were resentful, the Big Book suggests that the reason we are angry has do with incidents affecting us on a personal level, namely, "our self-esteem, our pocketbooks, our ambitions, our personal relationships (including sex) being hurt or threatened." These are what we write in the third column (Alcoholics Anonymous, 2001, p. 64-65).

What you are actually doing here is slowly moving the finger that points to others as the source of your discomfort, and pointing it to yourself. In this way, you begin to take responsibility for your own feelings. After all, how successful have you been at changing those with whom you have been resentful? You have probably not been very successful at all. Therefore, you have a choice. You can either sit around and stew about those you resent (and an alcoholic keeping a resentment often leads to relapse), or you can begin to change yourself and how you react to others. The Serenity Prayer, which is said at the end of many 12-Step meetings, addresses this point directly: "God, grant me the serenity to accept the things I cannot change, the courage to change the things I can, and the wisdom to know the difference" (Author Unknown). What you learn in your sobriety is that you cannot change most things outside of yourself. What you can change, with God's help, is you.

> "God, grant me the serenity to accept the things I cannot change, the courage to change the things I can, and the wisdom to know the difference" (Author Unknown).

Next comes the infamous fourth column. This will continue the process of pointing the finger at yourself. It calls for "disregard(ing) the other person involved entirely" (Alcoholics Anonymous, 2001, p. 67). You need to put on paper what you brought to the party

– what part you had in the situation that made you angry. This can be extremely difficult if you spent years blaming someone or something else for your resentments. You are now asked to turn your attention completely away from the other person and focus only on yourself. Remember, it is you, not the other person, who needs to change in order for you to get well.

At this point, a good question to again ask yourself is how badly do you want to get your life back. If you follow these steps, you will surely succeed at doing just that. If you balk at them, and think you have a better way, you will likely fail. Remember to employ Step 3 to gain the courage to take this honest look at yourself and take responsibility for your life.

Early on in sobriety, it was pointed out that most of the people whom I resented are much less affected by the resentment than I was. I had it in my mind that, by holding on to these resentments, I was punishing the other person. It was as if every time I thought of the incident, my anger was somehow causing them some pain or regret. The fact is that they don't have a clue when I'm thinking about it and it doesn't affect them in the least. So the only person who stays hurting is me! This awareness was very eye opening to me. All of the time and energy I put into such resentments was wasted. If that wasn't enough, it was also pointed out to me that the people whom I resent actually have power over me. Because of my distorted interpretation of what they did, I have this resentment which causes me much discomfort and keeps me sick. Now this really angered me. It was as if such people were allowed to occupy space in my head – rent-free! I remember saying to myself: "I'll be damned if I am going to allow this to happen!" I then became willing to proceed in the task at hand.

Step 4 also calls for identifying your fears and writing them down on paper (*Alcoholics Anonymous*, 2001, p. 68). This is an extremely important part of your inventory. Despite how well most alcoholics and addicts hide their fear from others, most have more fear than the normal population. The Big Book suggests that we are "driven by a hundred forms of fear" (*Alcoholics Anonymous*, 2001, p. 62). It manifests in various ways and is often hidden within other feelings such as anger and false pride. If fear is not acknowledged to yourself or others, it is often exhibited through other feelings.

In my experience, I developed a whole persona around such fear. This persona took the form of "Mr. Badass." I led everyone to believe that I was not somebody they wanted to mess with because, if they did, I would make them pay physically. I am not proud to say that I got into many fights proving this to be true. In fact, all people had to do was look at me wrong and I was in their face. The truth about this is that I was an absolute fraud. I was no tough guy. I was a scared little mouse doing whatever I could to survive in this world. It took the honesty of my 4th Step inventory to admit this and it was one of the turning points of my sobriety.

Finally, you must do a sexual inventory. "We reviewed our conduct over the years past. Where had we been selfish, dishonest, or inconsiderate? Whom had we hurt? Did we unjustifiably arouse jealousy, suspicion, or bitterness? Where were we at fault, what should we have done instead? We got this all down on paper and looked at it" (Alcoholics Anonymous, 2001, p. 69). This section may be especially difficult because you may be very ashamed sexually and want to take some of your secrets to the grave. Most sponsors will also share some of their secrets regarding their sexual past and this is very validating. You find out that you are not the freak you thought you were in regards to your sexual past. This step can also be very difficult because you may have "used" most of your partners or hurt them in some other way. This may be another eye-opener for you to discover how selfish you were in relationships.

There are many ways in which this step can be done. Each individual sponsor might suggest working it in a different way. Some utilize workbooks in which you list your resentments, fears, people you hurt, people who hurt you, things you are ashamed about, and examples of your false pride, shame, and sources of sadness in your life. Others have done it exactly the way the Big Book suggests. Remember, you select your sponsor because you want what he or she has. I suggest working this step the way your sponsor suggests because it is most likely the way your sponsor did it.

My first sponsor gave me a Step 4 workbook similar to the one just described and it was very effective for me. When I was five years sober, I decided my program needed a lift so I picked a man to be my sponsor who spoke of the value of working the steps exactly how the Big Book suggests working them. I followed his direction and that method was also of great benefit for me. I believe that God set it up so I got what I needed at every given point in my sobriety.

Step 5: Admitted to God, to ourselves, and to another human being the exact nature of our wrongs.

Now that you have written all of this down, it is time to share it with your Higher Power and another human being. I suggest sharing this with your sponsor, but it is not mandatory. Some people have done it with a priest or a trusted friend in the program. What is most important is that you are able to trust the person with your secrets. It is probably best to do it with your sponsor because it is preferable that your sponsor knows as much about you as possible. The more your sponsor knows about you, the better your sponsor is able to recognize when you are slipping back into old patterns.

When writing my Step 4, I was having a difficult time being completely honest because I was writing it in anticipation of having to share it with my sponsor. The problem was that the person I chose as a sponsor was the brother of a close friend of mine and I was hesitant to share everything with him. This could have been avoided by choosing a sponsor who was not a previous acquaintance. So it was suggested to me that I write the inventory as honestly as possible and then decide whom I would read it to. I did just that and made a decision to share it with a person in the program whom I had grown to trust and respect. This man shared openly in meetings some of the stuff I was uncomfortable sharing with anyone.

While sharing this inventory, it is important to be aware of God's presence because the step calls for us to "Admit to God... the exact nature of our wrongs." This step also calls for admitting wrongs to "ourselves" so it is also very important to listen to and understand your inventory as you are reading it. Sharing your inventory is difficult when you are doing it, but it is one of the most cleansing experiences you can have. Imagine sharing all this stuff with another human being and still being able to be accepted by that person. You end up feeling like you have no more skeletons in the closet. The effect is often very profound and it can be immediate, or realized over time.

Step 6: Were entirely ready to have God remove all these defects of character, and Step 7: Humbly asked Him to remove our short-comings.

Having shared your inventory, you will recognize things about you that don't look very attractive. You have acted against your morals and developed into a person you did not want to become. It is time to make a list of character defects that, if changed, will allow you to become the person you want to be. More importantly, it will allow you to become comfortable enough in your own skin to stay sober.

A good way to explore your character defects is to review your inventory with your sponsor. Your sponsor will probably point out some defects that you are not able to see. Again, honesty is essential in this step if you are to attain the maximum benefit the steps have to offer. Following are some common examples of character defects:

- Selfishness
- Self-centeredness
- Dishonesty
- Procrastination
- Quick temper
- Impatience
- Negativity
- Closed-mindedness
- Lust
- Self-pity
- Arrogance
- Being a phony
- Laziness

Once you have identified your character defects, you need to be willing to have God remove them *all*. In looking ahead at this step, I really thought it would be one of the easier ones. However, it turned out to be the most difficult step for me:

As mentioned earlier, I created a reputation for myself as being a tough guy. I actually started believing it myself. It worked well for me in keeping other people, especially men, at an emotional distance. It also worked as a protective mechanism to keep people from hurting me. Since this had become my identity, I was extremely fearful of who I would become without it. I thought I would become some kind of sissy. This fear was so great that I was not willing, at all, to have this character defect removed. In working with my sponsor on this issue, we agreed that, since I was not willing, I should begin praying for the willingness to become willing. I prayed on a daily basis for this willingness.

It all came to a head one night when I was pulling out of a parking lot onto the boulevard. I was turning right and I looked to my left for clearance and proceeded. Fortunately, I looked again as I was pulling out and had to slam on my brakes to avoid getting broad-sided by a guy driving a hot-rod going about 80 mph! As he went by, I started to give him "the finger" and suddenly remembered I was trying to work on that behavior and pulled my hand down. However, it was too late. He noticed what I had done and slammed on his brakes. Trying to avoid an altercation, I pulled into the next driveway hoping I could find refuge in a convenience store. It was my hope that I could walk into the store and he would go away. I was not so fortunate. He pulled in right behind me, got out of his car, and blocked my entrance into the store.

This was a very difficult situation for me because I would not normally think twice about "kicking his butt." Additionally, he was just the kind of guy I used to love to beat up – he was my size and he thought he was tough. But I had also agreed with my sponsor that I would avoid fighting at all cost. He began verbally assaulting me and I showed great restraint by remaining silent. I was taking personal responsibility for avoiding a fight and knew if I said anything, he would swing at me. Swallowing much pride and using all the self-control I could muster, I stated: "I don't want none of you, man" and turned my back on him and walked into the store. Fully expecting that he might "cold-cock" me from behind, I was very relieved when I turned around and he was walking away. I had done it! I walked away from a fight for the first time in my life!

I drove home to share the incident with my wife, but she was not home. As I sat home alone, my head turned on me and my "committee" began giving me uncomfortable thoughts. Instead of feeling proud of myself, there was a large part of me that felt I might have actually chickened out. If this wasn't difficult enough for me to take, the thought that the other guy may have thought the same thing was intolerable.

I became so uncomfortable with myself, I decided I had better attend a meeting despite having a severe cold. I shared about the incident, and my uncomfortable feelings, and began bawling my eyes out. Although the pain was very profound, simply sharing about it and experiencing the pain allowed me to get through it. I got plenty of positive strokes from my peers for what had happened and I felt very good when I left the group. Later that night, as I began my evening prayer routine, it occurred to me that if I was willing to do what I had done that night, I must be willing to have God remove my character defects. I got down on my knees at that moment, opened the Big Book, and said the 7th Step prayer. This was an extreme breakthrough for me and another turning point in my recovery. My willingness to change had risen to an all-time high. I might add that I rather like the person underneath that tough-guy mask.

Finally, in regard to Steps 6 and 7, for years in my recovery I had not realized how difficult it would be to shake my character defects. They had such a stranglehold on my life that I was not capable of removing them myself. After I had taken this step, I tried my hardest not to engage in them. I must tell you I failed miserably in many of them. Since I had, in a sense, made a pact with God that I would like to have them removed, it caused me much shame when I fell back into such defective behavior.

While in therapy, it was pointed out to me that I was approaching my character defects in the wrong way. I was reminded that the reason I needed to ask God to remove them was because I was incapable of removing them myself. This simple feedback has allowed me to view my shortcomings in a whole new light. I no longer have to feel ashamed when I fall short and I'm able to accept what my therapist affectionately calls: "My inner bastard." Nobody is perfect. I have certainly proven this over the years. So, instead of beating myself up when my inner bastard rears its ugly head, I can say to myself, "There it is, and that's why I need God's help."

Step 8: Made a list of all persons we had harmed, and became willing to make amends to them all.

Once you have taken a thorough inventory of yourself, have identified your character defects, and are praying to have them removed, it is then time to begin identifying those whom you have hurt in your life. So you put down on paper a list of your victims. For most alcoholics and addicts this list is quite extensive. Again, honesty with yourself is essential in working this step adequately. This process is uncomfortable and it feels like you are dredging up parts of your past that would be better left alone. However, you must proceed if you are to fully recover. You are very much affected by the pain you have caused others and you cannot repress the truth about yourself any longer if you expect to remain sober. As you did in the fourth column of your inventory, it is best to disregard the other person's involvement entirely. After all, it is you who needs to change – not others. You are going to clean up your side of the street.

Once you have completed your list, the next part of the step is to become "willing to make amends to them *all.*" You cannot say to yourself, "Okay. I'm willing to make amends to everyone but my ex-wife (or ex-husband)." It is important that you achieve willingness to clean up your whole mess, not just part of it. No matter how strong your past resentments have been, you need to get humble enough to clean up your side of the street. By making amends, you are not making a statement that anything bad they did is all right with you. You are simply making amends for your part in it. You will leave it up to the other person to clean up their own mess if they decide to do so. If not, that's on them. You have taken care of yourself and that is what you are told will make you better.

If the resentment still keeps you from becoming willing to make amends to someone you resent, you might want to begin praying for that person. The Big Book states: "We realized that the people who had wronged us were perhaps spiritually sick. Though we did not like their symptoms and the way these disturbed us, they, like ourselves, were sick too. We asked God to help us show them the same tolerance, pity, and patience that we would cheerfully grant a sick friend. When a person offended we said to ourselves, 'This is a sick man. How can I be helpful to him? God save me from being angry. Thy will be done'" (Alcoholics Anonymous, 2001, pp. 66-67). So you pray for this individual just as you would pray for a sick friend.

This has been a very valuable tool in my own recovery. After I had completed my 5th Step, my sponsor had me make a list of those I still resented and pray for them daily. One by one, I was able to take these people off my list until, amazingly, nobody remained on it. Being persistent in my prayer for an offender allowed the resentment to slowly slip away. It makes sense that if you are trying to pray away a resentment, one of two things will eventually happen. Either you will stop praying, or you will stop resenting. The two cannot co-exist for long.

Step 9: Made direct amends to such people wherever possible, except when to do so would injure them or others.

Now you are ready to clean up your side of the street. You make amends to every person on your list. You apologize for your actions and ask if there is anything you can do to make things better. Often there are financial amends necessary and these must be corrected. If you owe money, you need to make things right by being financially responsible for your wrongs.

When making amends, you do not attempt to justify your behavior. You simply state what you have done wrong and apologize for it. No matter the reaction you get, you do not engage in a debate with them. You own your behavior and do not bring up how they have wronged you. It is very important to know you are not necessarily

> All you are doing is apologizing and offering to make things right. Their acceptance of your apology is not required.

seeking their forgiveness. Although this is nice when it happens, it is not a determinant of your success on this step. All you are doing is apologizing and offering to make things right. *Their acceptance of your apology is not required.* You are simply doing all *you* can.

In my experience, most of the amends went quite well. Many of the people were hearing me take ownership of my behavior, without blaming anyone or anything, for the very first time. They seemed to appreciate that. They were usually very happy that I was finally doing something about my problem.

It is at this point, the following "promises" of the program begin to become reality:

> "If we are painstaking about this phase of our development, we will be amazed before we are half way through (Step 9). We are going to know a new freedom and a new happiness. We will not regret the past nor wish to shut the door on it. We will comprehend the word serenity and we will know peace. No matter how far down the scale we have gone, we will see how our experience can benefit others. That feeling of uselessness and self-pity will disappear. We will lose interest in selfish things and gain interest in our fellows. Self-seeking will slip away. Our whole attitude and outlook upon life will change. Fear of people and of economic insecurity will leave us. We will intuitively know how to handle situations which used to baffle us. We will suddenly realize that God is doing for us what we could not do for ourselves. Are these extravagant promises? We think not. They are being fulfilled among us – sometimes quickly, sometimes slowly. They will always materialize if we work for them" (Alcoholics Anonymous, 2001, pp 83-84).

As a result of working steps 4 through 9, you have completed a rigorous moral inventory and pulled the skeletons out of your closet, identified your character defects and have asked God to remove them, and have made amends to everyone in your life whom you have harmed. You have removed the obstacles to doing what you decided to do in Step 3 – to turn your will and life over to God. What an absolute freeing feeling this is! Just think about it. All that stuff you used to stew about and/or beat yourself up over is gone! All that stuff that got in the way of getting closer to a Higher Power has been removed. If I could just share with you what it feels like to be on this side of the steps, you would surely follow this path – I hope you do.

Step 10: Continued to take personal inventory and when we were wrong promptly admitted it.

Once you have cleaned house, Step 10 is designed to keep it clean. At the end of your day, you review what ways you may have gone against your morals, what character defects you have engaged in, and whom have you hurt through your actions that day. If there is anything to clean up, you do so quickly. As it states in the Big Book, you continue to pray to have your character defects removed and plan to make amends to anyone you have harmed (Alcoholics Anonymous, 2001, p. 84). In this way, you keep the slate clean and, thus, feel good about yourself and enhance your chances at staying sober. Without this step, you would build up a whole new inventory. Following is an example of how the 10th step can be done:

My current sponsor, Bob S., has me do a daily 10th step that I find particularly effective. First thing in the morning, after I read my morning meditation passage, I address the fears I identified in my 4th Step by saying a modified 3rd Step prayer: "God, I offer myself to you – to build with me and to do with me as you wilt. Relieve me of the bondage of self, that I may better do your will. Take away my difficulties, (insert fears here) that victory over them may bear witness to those I would help of your Power, your Love, and your Way of Life. May I do your will always!" (Alcoholics Anonymous, 2001, p. 63). I follow this with a prayer similar to the example I shared earlier in which I attempt to "turn it over."

At night, I review my day and explore the possibility of any new resentment. If so, I write the name down and pray for that person just as I do anyone else who might remain on my list. The prayer goes like this: "God, grant the following people happiness, joy, and peace: (insert names here). Don't let me hold any anger, hatred, or resentment towards any of these people and, if I have harmed them in any way, forgive me and let their lives be whole, happy, and complete."

I then take an honest look at how I did regarding my character defects. I identify those areas in which I fell short and say a modified 7th Step prayer: "My Creator, I am now willing that you should have all of me, good and bad. I pray that you now remove from me every single de-

fect of character (insert character defects here) which stands in the way of my usefulness to you and to my fellows. Grant me strength, as I go out from here, to do your bidding. Amen" (Alcoholics Anonymous, 2001, p. 76).

Finally, I review my day to check if I owe anyone amends due to my behavior that day. If I do, I make a plan to make the amends as soon as possible.

In this way, you can keep the slate clean and attain that cleansing feeling you attained by working the previous steps. I can't express to you the freedom and serenity this provides you by waking up every morning knowing that you are being accountable and doing everything you can to be the person you want to be, and more importantly, who God wants you to be!

Step 11: Sought through prayer and meditation to improve our conscious contact with God *as we understood Him*, praying only for knowledge of His will for us and the power to carry that out.

Once you have removed what gets in the way of turning your will and life over to your Higher Power, you can move directly toward seeking knowledge of what your God wants and becoming a vehicle for His will. This is done by praying for such knowledge regularly and meditating for the answer God has for you. This will, in effect, allow you to focus less on what you want and more on what God wants. As seen in Chapter 4, you may choose to believe that prayer is talking to God, and meditation is listening to God. The key to meditation, or listening to God, is to quiet your thoughts down enough to allow God to speak to you. Here are some meditation techniques that are particularly effective.

Breathing exercises are known to be useful in meditation. In *Relapse Prevention for Addictive Behaviors* (1990), Wanigaratne, Wallace, Pullin, Keany, and Farmer suggest a good one in which you do the following: breathe in while counting to ten; wait before exhaling while counting to ten; exhale while counting to ten; and waiting before taking your next breath while counting to ten (p. 75). The speed in which you count should be adjusted so you can do it comfortably without hyperventilating and ensuring you get enough air. Focusing on breathing and counting enables you to clear your head of the stressors in your life. Once you have done the exercise for about five minutes, you can then shift your focus onto your Higher Power. Since you are trying to give up your will for what your God wants, you attempt to listen to what your Higher Power wants to tell you. "The answers will come if your own house is in order" (Alcoholics Anonymous, 2001, p. 164) – and your house should be in order as you have done the housecleaning in Steps 4 – 9 and are keeping it clean with Step 10. If your mind drifts while focusing on your Higher Power, start the breathing exercise again until your head clears. Then put your focus again on what your God wants for you.

My favorite meditation technique is one I learned when I was in the seventh grade. I was amazed at the comfort level and serenity this method produced. I was asked to close my eyes and imagine that lukewarm water was slowly moving up my body. I imagined the water slowly moving over my toes, the arch of my foot, my heels, up to and over my ankle, up my calf, and toward and over my knees. At this point, I was asked to imagine that, from the knees down, I was weightless – as if they were floating in water. I then continued by imagining the water moving up my thighs, toward and over my buttocks and over my waist. Again, I was asked to take an inventory of my body ensuring that the lower part of my body felt like it was floating. This inventory included focusing on each before-mentioned body part. I then imagined the water moving up my stomach and lower back, up toward my chest, and up to and over my shoulders. At this point, I was instructed that my shoulders should feel like they are dropping in relaxation. Again, I took inventory to ensure that each body part felt like it was floating. Finally, I imagined the water moving up my neck, toward my chin and the back of my head, up my cheek, over my nose, to my eyes, up my forehead, and eventually, covering my entire body. Again, I took an inventory of my body to ensure that I felt completely relaxed as if my whole body was floating in water. This technique worked very well and I became more relaxed than I had ever been in my life.

In using this technique today, the extended focus on relaxing my body allows me to clear my head and listen for God's will for me. My focus is exclusively on God's will. If my mind drifts from my intended focus,

I simply go back through the exercise or simply take inventory of my body's relaxation level to, once again, clear my head. I also found a breathing technique that enables me to keep my focus on God. I imagine that, when I breathe in, I am breathing in my Higher Power or all that is good. When I exhale, I imagine that I am breathing out the disease or all that is bad or impure. This has been a great way of staying focused on my Higher Power during meditation and it is very cleansing.

Don't be discouraged if you don't feel you're doing it right. If you are persistent in practicing meditation, even if it's only 10 minutes a day, it will become much more comfortable. You will get increasingly better at clearing your head and the answers from your Higher Power will come. As self-centered as most alcoholics and addicts are, even if you don't feel like you are receiving answers right away, just getting out of your head and temporarily shutting off your wants and needs is a move in the right direction.

Your Step 11 prayer and meditation should be done on a daily basis in order to grow in your spirituality. As you progress in working Step 11, you are provided with increasingly more insight regarding what God wants you to do. It also allows you to achieve the peace of mind resulting from the acknowledgment that your Higher Power is in control. This is a far cry from the focus that most of us have had in attempting to achieve our own ends. It takes the daily focus on Step 11 to continue to move toward God's ends.

In the discussion on Step 3 earlier in this chapter, I mentioned that I start my day by attempting to turn my will and life over to God as the step indicates. Typically, this only lasts until I allow the stresses of daily life to take over and begin believing again that I am ultimately responsible for what happens in God's world. I then come to my senses, recognize that I am Edging God Out (how do you like that acronym?) and attempt to turn my will back over to God. When I do this, I attain a very high degree of serenity by realizing that I am simply re-

sponsible for the "foot-work" toward what I believe God wants in His world and that He, alone, is responsible for the results. This is possible for self-centered people like us and, prior to sobriety, I could never have imagined the serenity this way of life provides.

Step 12: Having had a spiritual awakening as the result of these steps, we tried to carry this message to alcoholics, and to practice these principles in all our affairs.

As the beginning of this step implies, the result of working the first eleven steps is a spiritual awakening. You will not view the world the same. You will see the world with what Dr. Paul calls, "a new pair of glasses" (Alcoholics Anonymous, 2001, p. 418). Your view of the world will be spiritually influenced rather than by selfish interests. Most of us who have arrived at this point are more than happy to pass this way of life on to other alcoholics. It is as if the excitement of our personal transformation simply won't allow us to keep it to ourselves.

However, this is not the main reason you pass it on. You must help other alcoholics in order to stay sober. It is a matter of saving your own butt. One of the reasons this works is that it gets you out of yourself. If you are like most alcoholics, you have a tendency to be very self-centered and only concerned with what you can get out of life. When

> You must help other alcoholics in order to stay sober.

you don't get what you want, you feel deprived and resentful. Helping others allows you to defocus on what *you* should be getting out of life and start caring about *others*.

Another reason this works is that helping others usually results in hearing how bad the newcomer's life is which reminds you of where you came from. Additionally, passing on the solution requires you to revisit what you've done in order to progress in your recovery. These are both valuable pieces of information to revisit so you can continue to take the steps necessary to avoid going back to where you were.

As mentioned earlier, the fellowship of AA was founded on this basis. Bill W. and Dr. Bob wondered how they would keep their sobriety and eventually realized that it was helping others that kept them sober. Helping others can include: sponsorship; participating in 12-Step panels, in which each panelist shares his or her story to fellow alcoholics/addicts in a hospital or institution; telling one's story at a 12-Step meeting; making 12th Step calls in which an alcoholic/addict visits another at his home, in a hospital, or elsewhere and shares his or her experience, strength, and hope; or simply putting one's hand out at a meeting to greet a newcomer.

Finally, 12-Step principles are practiced "in all our affairs." You must "walk the talk." If you are working Steps 10 and 11 on a daily basis, this part of Step 12 comes natural. You are facing your behavior on a daily basis and attempting to live the life you feel that God wants you to live.

It is my hope that this review of the 12 Steps has both enlightened you and provided hope that you no longer have to live uncomfortably in your own skin. I must tell you that when I received this information, I was quite skeptical and fearful that I could not actually achieve what those before me had achieved through these steps. What it did provide me was a level of hope that enabled me to go through with it. Much to my delight and relief, it worked. My life has not been the same since. I sincerely hope you give it a try. I have never heard of anyone being disappointed with the results of working these steps.

CHAPTER 7
DEALING WITH FEELINGS

A s mentioned earlier, we alcoholics and addicts appear to be inherently sensitive people. We seem to worry more than normal people do. To accentuate this hypersensitivity, we are also very intolerant of emotion. Our first instinct when we get an emotion is to run from it. Hence, the primary reason we abuse substances is to suppress our feelings. Additionally, the more emotions we suppress through our chemical use, the more chemicals are necessary to keep them at bay.

A popular opinion is that in order for people to recover, they need to resolve issues that lead to uncomfortable emotions. This opinion is somewhat warranted, however, I believe the resolution of issues is secondary to learning how to feel and tolerate uncomfortable emotion. One might be able to resolve some issues that lead to uncomfortable feelings but, since life is full of such issues, learning to tolerate emotion is paramount. Additionally, if we learn to feel our emotions while working a program of recovery for support, their intensity will gradually diminish. I call this "mastering emotions."

> ...resolution of issues is secondary to learning how to feel, and tolerate uncomfortable emotion.

Alcoholics and addicts are slaves to emotion. When uncomfortable emotion arises, it takes control by leading us to our drug of choice and the inherent consequences. No matter how much we want to avoid this behavior, we have no choice – we simply can't tolerate the discomfort of our emotion. In this way emotions are our masters. In order for us to be free of this enslavement, we must master our emotions. This is done by embracing rather than running from them. After all, emotions are God-given. They are normal, and humans are supposed to have them. When you experience an emotion, your attitude needs to be, "Well, here's another one of those uncomfortable emotions. It looks like I'm going to have to feel this for a while, so I'd better contact my sober support system and my Higher Power so I can get through this." As you work your program of recovery and experience the emotion, it becomes more tolerable and has increasingly less power over you. Eventually, this particular emotion loses its intensity and you no longer have a need to run from it.

> As you work your program of recovery and experience the emotion, it becomes more tolerable and has increasingly less power over you.

Therefore, the emotion no longer has power over you and, thus, you have "mastered" that particular emotion. As you move along in your recovery and practice experiencing your emotions with help from your sober support system, you no longer go into panic when one hits because you know you have tools of recovery to get through it.

In my drinking and using career, whenever an emotion arose, my attitude was, "Boy, this is lousy. I'm not going to sit here and feel this. I'm getting the heck out of here!" I then proceeded to get loaded. Upon entry into recovery, I would often complain at meetings about how strong and intolerable the emotions were. My drama was apparent as I made a really big deal about it. I expected the reaction of others to be more in line with mine – to act like it was a big deal. Rather, the reaction sounded to me like, "Big deal. So you have an emotion." At one such time, a member of the group asked, "Can you just make it okay to feel lousy once in a while?" I was flabbergasted! That notion had never occurred to me. It helped me to be less reactive to emotion and just make it okay to feel. I still took the action that was suggested to me, but my initial reaction to emotion became much tamer. It caused me to be much less resentful as I worked the tools of recovery to get through the uncomfortable feeling.

At this point, let's take a brief look at some of the emotions that cause so much discomfort.

Shame

When you feel shame, you feel like you just don't measure up. At its extreme, you feel absolutely worthless – that your existence has no meaning and it was a mistake to put you on this earth. You feel inferior and have a tendency to seek approval from others so you can feel good about yourself. When you don't receive such validation, you take it as further evidence that you are worthless.

Many people equate shame with guilt. These two feelings are somewhat similar, but there are distinctions between the two. Guilt is the feeling you get when you *do* something bad, and shame is the uncomfortable feeling you get when you feel you *are* bad. Shame often arises when you do bad things and feel that, as a result, you are a bad person. An effective way to combat shame that arises in this way is to recognize you are imperfect and you make mistakes. It doesn't mean you are a bad person, it means you are a normal person. Everyone makes mistakes. It is human nature. God made us that way – imperfect. If you were perfect, you would be some kind of freak. Therefore, if God made us imperfect, and you are imperfect, then you are normal. The fact that you are imperfect actually makes you a perfect creation of God. Therefore, you are perfectly imperfect!

Many people have deep-rooted shame that stems from childhood messages. If you consistently received messages as a child that you don't measure up, you will grow up believing it. In this way, shame has its roots in low self-esteem. When you have low self-esteem, you have a low opinion of yourself. When you get messages from your environment that you don't measure up, no matter how minute the message might be, you take it as further proof of your unworthiness. This belief that you are not okay is so deep-rooted that evidence to the contrary is often ignored. The negative cues from your environment are given more attention than the positive ones. Consequently, when you *make* a mistake, you end up feeling like you *are* a mistake.

This was especially true in my own pre-recovery and early recovery. If I was in a room full of people and had the approval of everyone except for one person, it was that one person on whom I would focus. It didn't matter that I had a 90% approval rating; I focused on that one person as further proof of my inadequacy. In order for me to feel good about myself, I would need to turn that person around about me and I would often set about doing just that.

As mentioned above, the strategy in surviving feelings in early recovery is learning to tolerate them. Shame is no different. You must work your program and gain support from your peers and Higher Power so you can master your shame instead of being controlled by it. Your sober support system will help you challenge the negative messages you give yourself. Over time, you will begin to be reconditioned by positive messages that challenge the negatives you latch onto. Additionally, through working the steps, you begin to build self-esteem so shame is less likely to surface. This self-esteem building is extremely important in recovery, and now I want to share with you some of my experience in building self-esteem.

Building Self-esteem

I will start by letting you know that I had a very difficult childhood with a father who was extremely strict. He had a violent temper and often hit me much harder than any child should be hit. At the time, I felt this was normal and I'm sure Dad meant no malice, as I believed this was the way he was treated by his alcoholic father. In one such instance, I woke up in the middle of the night and he was beating me. I don't remember if I knew then what the beating was about, but it sure didn't do much for my self-esteem.

I could never really live up to my father's expectations despite seeking his approval constantly. Mom always gave me strong emotional support and often went overboard – I think to make up for my Dad's lack of approval. It just wasn't enough, however, and the only thing I can figure is that my father was my male role model and I needed his approval more. It was very rare that I ever received positive feedback from Dad and the negative feedback was abundant. When I failed at something, or did not live up to his expectations, I was ridiculed and/or yelled at. When I succeeded at something or felt that I had met his expectations, I was treated as though it was simply what was expected, rather than something that should be praised.

On one occasion, Dad and my three younger brothers were sitting in the living room, and for reasons unknown to me, Dad proceeded to let us know what he thought we would be when we grew up. Starting with my younger brothers, he stated that one would be a doctor, another a lawyer, and the last would be an entertainer. Then he got to me and stated that he thought I would be a trash collector. What is a ten-year-old boy supposed to do with this information? I was definitely hurt by this, but not so surprised because I felt this was really what he thought about me. This was based on the negative messages I consistently received from him. This drove me all the more to try to prove to him that I was not worthless and to try to make him proud. I regretfully spent my whole childhood trying to meet his unreachable expectations of me. I believe this also continued into adulthood as I worked in the family printing business for fifteen years in a job that I hated. In therapy, during my recovery, I came to the conclusion that I probably worked for him for so long because I figured he would not consider me as a trash collector and I would eventually make him proud by doing what he did for a living.

Since trying to reach Dad's unreachable expectations continued into adulthood, it seemed that his unreachable expectations of me turned into my unreachable expectations of me. I could never be satisfied with anything I achieved. I would set my sights on a goal, and when it was reached, I would not be satisfied and would raise the bar. I would then achieve that goal, and being unsatisfied, I would raise the bar again. I strongly believe that the low self-esteem resulting from the negative feedback I received as a child is the cause of my perfectionism into adulthood – a trait I continue to struggle with occasionally.

Self-esteem is esteem that comes from within. If you have low self-esteem, good feelings about yourself do not come from you. Therefore, you seek esteem elsewhere – from your environment. You become a people-pleaser to get positive strokes from others so you can feel good about yourself. You base how you feel about yourself on what other people think about you. If you do not have the approval of others, you feel lousy about yourself and experience shame as a result. You become a social chameleon as you change your colors according to your environment. You act one way around a certain group of people because you think acting that way will get their approval. You then act completely different around another group so as to get their approval. The problem with this is you become completely dependent on others to feel good about yourself. You have no identity because you wear masks hiding who you really are. You do this so you can be who you think others want you to be and to attain the positive strokes that will make you feel worthwhile. Here are some of the things I do that you can use to improve your self-esteem. Try them so you will feel more at ease with yourself.

The "Bob Filter"

When I became a counselor, I struggled with allowing feedback from other people to mean so much to me. A client might say to me, "Bob, I did not approve of the way you handled that group. I felt that you spent too much time dealing with Joe's problems and should have given other members more of a chance." When I received such feedback, I felt devastated and that the group had finally "found me out" – that I have no business being a counselor. On the other hand, someone in the group might tell me, "Bob, that was a great group. You are a wonderful counselor and I'm happy to be in your group." With this information, I would become ecstatic. I felt I had finally "arrived" as a counselor and I really belonged in this profession.

I overcame this problem by creating what I call the "Bob Filter." This filter allows me to immediately check out any feedback with myself before reacting to it internally. It works something like this. If someone gives me the above negative feedback, I say to myself, "Hmm. This person thinks I did a lousy job in group." I would then evaluate this information myself to determine whether or not I agreed with it. I might say to myself, "Well, I guess I have to agree with this person because I really didn't feel like I was pumping on all cylinders and I admittedly did not have a good group. But everyone has a bad group every once in a while, so I'll only allow myself to feel moderately bad." This is a far cry from the devastation I felt and the questioning of whether or not I belonged in this profession. Conversely, I might say to myself, "Hmm. This person thinks I did a lousy job in group. I guess I have to disagree with this person regarding my performance because I actually think I did a great job in there and that it was just what I think that group needed. I'm sorry this person feels I did a lousy job in group, but I cannot allow myself to feel bad as a result of someone else's opinion. In fact, I'm going to allow myself to feel good about that group because I believe I did a good job."

If I am going to use the Bob Filter for negative feedback, I also need to use it for positive feedback. If someone says to me, "Bob, I think you did a great job in that group," I would again check it out with myself to see how I felt about it." I might say to myself, "Hmm. This person thinks I did a good job in that group. However, I didn't feel like I did that great of a job. In fact, I think this was actually one of my off nights. It's cool that this person thinks I did a good job, but I have to disagree so I'm not going to allow myself to feel too good about it." Conversely, I might say to myself, "Hmm. This person thinks I did a good job in that group. You know what? I have to agree. I think I did an excellent job in that group so I'm going to go ahead and allow myself to feel pretty good about it." Again, this is much different than allowing myself to be ecstatic about myself based on feedback from another.

Through the use of the Bob Filter, I am no longer controlled by the feedback of others. I now feel about myself based on what *I* think about me, rather than on what *others* think about me. My esteem now comes from within – hence, I have self-esteem.

Pointing the Headlights In

In therapy, I shared my tendency to care too much about what other people think about me. My therapist suggested my problem was related to spending too much time focused on my environment and not enough time focused on myself. He stated that I had "headlights" which were constantly pointed outward looking toward my environment and I needed to get the headlights pointed inward. I found this to be absolutely true and gained insight into the fact that everything I did had the purpose of gaining some type of response from others. I found it amazing that nothing I ever did was truly for me and how I would make myself feel. Needless to say, this was unacceptable to me and I wanted to make a change. My therapist suggested that I spend nine minutes a day alone and totally focused on myself. He told me this might be difficult at first so I should start by simply focusing on my body and my basic needs. I gave this a try and sat in a chair actually looking down at my body and concentrating on it. I next focused on my basic needs and asked myself if I was hungry, thirsty, tired, etc. He was right. It was extremely difficult at first to focus on myself because I had never done that. It eventually became a little more comfortable and, on subsequent days, I began focusing on my wants. I asked myself what I wanted out of life and spent a few sittings just thinking about that. I next focused on my values, and finally my strengths. This strategy worked very well for me. As a result of spending so much time focused on myself, I actually started to attain an identity. Imagine that. I actually began to identify the guy who was underneath all those masks.

Private Goal-setting

I also dealt with my tendency to seek the approval of my supervisors, peers, and even clients. My therapist suggested that I set three goals every day I went to work. I would then try to achieve these goals without telling anyone about them. At the end of the day, I was to evaluate how I did on achieving these goals. I would then base how I felt about my performance on how I did on them. In this way, I was able to base my feelings on what I thought about me rather than on what others thought about me. Again, my esteem started to come from within rather than from without. This provided me with much freedom in life and I began feeling genuinely good about myself.

Other Self-esteem Building Tools

My therapist also suggested that, since I never do anything without seeking the approval of others, I should do something good for someone and not tell anyone about it. This also worked to build self-esteem because the good feeling I received from such action came from me alone.

I might add here that working the steps is also a very good way to build self-esteem. This is especially true with Steps 4 through 10 as we focus on ourselves and clean the slate. I also want to suggest a book that aided me in building self-esteem. It was introduced to me by a friend and mentor who was also my professor in college. She felt it was very important that addiction professionals attain some personal growth and self-esteem. The book is called: *How Do I Love Me* and was written by Helen M. Johnson (1986). In the book, Johnson has the reader focus on such areas as attitude, strengths, values, perfectionism, a personal support system, and goal setting. This book is not very lengthy and gets right to the point in building self-esteem. I strongly encourage you to begin taking steps to build your self-esteem and you will eventually find you have much less shame.

Humility vs. Grandiosity

The term *humility* is defined in *Webster's Dictionary* (1979) as "a state or quality of being humble of mind or spirit" (p. 884). *Humble* is defined as "having or showing a consciousness of one's defects or shortcomings" (p. 884). Many in the program speak of the importance of humility in recovery. It takes humility to be honest about who you are. If you can do that, you can begin to *accept* yourself for who you are. Accepting yourself, shortcomings and all, will result in a decrease in the amount of shame you feel. Just as important is that if you can be humble enough to be honest with others about your shortcomings and difficulties, you can receive their help and support. How can anyone help you if you can't acknowledge a need for it?

Although having humility in the program is important, it is often a difficult quality to learn – especially for alcoholics and addicts. The problem is that, when you allow others to see your shortcomings – and God knows most alcoholics and addicts are not used to doing this – it may result in shame. You have spent your drinking and using careers avoiding such emotional pain. When you stop using, it is hard enough just dealing with the shame that comes up in daily life. Now you are being asked to get humble which directly evokes more shame. Additionally, since alcoholics and addicts often have very strong egos, they don't want others to see their vulnerability. They wear a mask that states to others, "Everything is okay with me. I'm just fine." This mask is known as "grandiosity." Are you wearing this mask?

In early recovery, many alcoholics and addicts avoid shame-evoking humility by engaging in grandiose behavior. In its mild form, grandiosity manifests as a denial that you have any problems. It can sound something like, "I'm just fine over here, and I really don't need your help." In its extreme form, one may become very arrogant and pompous: "I'm not only just fine, I'm actually better than all of you. There is nothing you have that I want." Notice the stark contrast between this attitude and the attitude of the humble person who is able to acknowledge his or her shortcomings and the need for help. Therefore, I propose that humility and grandiosity are at opposite ends of a continuum:

Figure 2

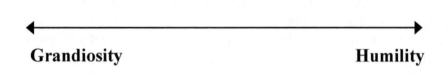

Grandiosity   **Humility**

The tendency to escape the shame associated with humility, by engaging in grandiose behavior, is further evidence of the importance of learning to tolerate the emotion of shame. Learning to live with such emotions is accomplished through the support of your sober support system.

While working in treatment, after educating my clients on the importance of dealing with shame rather than running from it, I will often have them write ten examples of shame in their lives. They share this list in group and receive support and validation from their peers. This assignment begins the process of desensitizing the impact of shame on their lives so they can tolerate future shame. Afterward, when shame arises in their daily lives, they remember that it is a feeling that they can experience and master with the support of others. They learn that instead of going into panic when shame arises, they can make a phone call to their sponsor or other member of their sober support system to attain the support they need to feel the feeling and get through it. I would recommend a similar assignment to be done with a therapist or in a therapy group. The main point here is that, instead of running from shame, it should be embraced as a natural human emotion that can be processed and worked through with the loving help of your sober support system.

Anger

Learning how to manage your anger is vital in recovery. When you got angry in the past, you probably ran straight to your drug of choice. Unless you learn to manage your anger in other ways, you will surely do the same thing no matter how much you want to stay sober. Aside from the fact that your anger gets so overwhelming that you don't know what else to do with it, you often get a case of the "screw-its." You say, "screw everything, and I don't care what the consequences are – I'm getting loaded." You often drink or use to hurt the person you are angry at – as if you are actually hurting the other person more than you are hurting yourself.

Another important reason for managing anger is that it often turns to resentment. As I quoted the Big Book earlier, "Resentment is the 'number one' offender. It destroys more alcoholics than anything else" (Alcoholics Anonymous, 2001, p. 64). The Big Book further emphasizes the danger of resentment:

> "It is plain that a life which includes deep resentment leads only to futility and unhappiness. ...with the alcoholic, whose hope is the maintenance and growth of a spiritual experience, this business of resentment is infinitely grave. We found that it is fatal. For when harboring such feelings we shut ourselves off from the sunlight of the Spirit. The insanity of alcohol returns and we drink again. And with us, to drink is to die. If we were to live, we had to be free of anger. The grouch and the brainstorm were not for us. They may be the dubious luxury of normal men, but for alcoholics these things are poison" (Alcoholics Anonymous, 2001, p. 66).

In case you miss the point here, what this tells us is that ridding ourselves of anger and resentment is not just something we think is a good idea for people in recovery, it is life and death for us. Normal people don't necessarily have to act accordingly –

...ridding ourselves of anger and resentment is not just something we think is a good idea for people in recovery, it is life and death for us.

their lives don't depend on it. Ours do, so we have no choice. Resentment goes beyond the acute feeling of anger. It occurs when you are unwilling to move beyond your anger and hold onto it over the long term. You refuse to forgive the person who makes you angry as if you are actually punishing the other person by holding onto it. You stew on the issue much harder and for longer periods of time than the person you are angry at. Remember that you are not hurting the other person by holding on to your resentment. The only person you are hurting with such resentment is yourself – especially since your resentment is dangerous to your sobriety.

As mentioned earlier, this fact was a great motivator for me to work Step 4 and to learn to manage my anger so further resentment would not develop. Let us now explore some ways of managing your anger. Notice that many of the anger management skills are simply ingredients for recovery being applied to anger.

Anger Management Tools

Call your sponsor

This is a great tool for managing anger because alcoholics and addicts usually get much angrier than the situation calls for. Your sponsor can help you identify this.

How this worked for me is that I would call my sponsor and let him know how angry I was. He would ask what makes me so angry and I proceeded to inform him of the impropriety that was inflicted. As I shared what happened, I found myself embellishing the story in an attempt to make the situation justify how angry I was. I would usually catch myself doing this and pull my own covers by suggesting to my sponsor that I was much angrier than the situation called for. Of course, my sponsor always agreed with this assessment. This simple recognition would calm me down and my sponsor and I would often end up laughing at my continued tendency to blow things out of proportion. Even in the times when I wasn't able to see my overreaction, just sharing my anger with another human being would have a calming effect.

The more you share your feelings, the less power they have over you. For this reason, **calling a sober peer** and **sharing at meetings** are also valuable anger management tools to help you in maintaining sobriety.

Journal writing

Writing about your anger is also very helpful because it allows you to feel the anger rather than run from it. It also gives you clarity regarding what your anger is all about.

In early recovery, I would usually start off on the first page by cursing that which made me angry. At this stage, the pen often penetrated through the page because I was so furious. In this way, I was able to express my anger without hurting anyone or anything, and not making a fool of myself – none of which I succeeded in doing in my using days.

Once I started calming down, I would explore on paper what it was about the situation that made me so angry. I usually came to the conclusion that the anger resulted from other feelings such as fear, hurt, helplessness, shame, guilt, or sadness. These feelings are very uncomfortable for me to feel. In fact, of all of the feelings I experience, I believe I am most comfortable with anger. This is most likely due to the fact that, with anger, I can externalize the issue onto someone or something other than myself. It is much easier to be angry at something or someone than to look at myself. Therefore, I run from other uncomfortable emotions by getting angry. I believe that anger is often a secondary emotion to other emotions. This is why the 4th Step inventory is so effective.

Through such journaling, you can discover what other emotions you might be running from by getting angry. This will allow you to calm down and deal with whatever emotion is underneath the anger and stop being so angry and resentful.

Work a Mini 4th Step

Remember from our earlier discussion on the 4th Step that you begin by writing the three columns: what or who makes you angry, the cause of your anger, and what it affects in you, i.e. "our self-esteem, our pocketbooks, our ambitions, or our personal or sexual relationships" (Alcoholics Anonymous, 2001, pp. 64-65). You then write a fourth column in which you explore what your part is in the situation. In this way, you get the focus off of what you are angry about and get focused on yourself. Remember, you have little or no control over the behavior of others and it is you who needs to change if you are to get well. When you get focused on yourself, the anger typically subsides.

> Remember, you have little or no control over the behavior of others and it is you who needs to change if you are to get well.

Exercise

It takes much energy to build up and maintain anger. It often seems as if you cannot gain relief from anger until you can expend some of the energy that goes into it.

When I lacked appropriate ways of releasing this energy, I got relief by hurting someone or breaking something. As mentioned previously, I regret the fact that there were many victims of my anger expression, which resulted in physical violence in my using days. I have since found that exercise works just as well in releasing the energy that goes into my anger. One way I do this is by getting on the ground and doing some angry push-ups. I do them fast and hard until I can do no more. I, effectively, expend all the energy I have for that moment and attain some level of satisfaction by doing so. In this way, I expend the energy that goes into my anger and I haven't hurt anybody or anything in the process. I believe any type of aerobic exercise will have the same effect. I have also gone out to the driving range to hit golf balls or to the batting cage to hit the ball as hard as I can. I know some people who hit a punching bag to expend their angry energy. I've also heard that kicking pillows works well.

Yell Inconspicuously

Another way of expending the energy that goes into your anger is to yell. In the past, you might have targeted someone with your yelling and, as a result, hurt someone or made a fool of yourself. Yelling into a pillow is an effective way of releasing your angry energy without having a victim. Another way is to turn your stereo up very loud and yell. By doing this you can also get it out without hurting anyone or drawing negative attention to yourself.

Sing or Whistle

Singing or whistling appears to work very well in calming an angry person down. For whatever reason, it is very hard to be angry and to sing or whistle at the same time.

I remember one time I walked into a supermarket and was in a very angry mood. I came across a transient-looking gentleman who was whistling away very contentedly. Here I was, running my own treatment center, making decent money, happily married with children, physically healthy, a homeowner, driving a decent car, and had many friends. I compared my situation to this man's who appeared to have very little. I had everything to be happy about, but was very discontent. This other guy had very little and probably much more to complain about. Yet, he was whistling away with, seemingly, not a care in the world. I asked myself, "What is wrong with this picture?" So I took up his cue and began whistling myself. The effect was very profound as my attitude lightened up almost immediately.

Pray or Meditate

As stated earlier, when you are discontent, you are basically saying that you know better than God does about what He should be doing in His world (Alcoholics Anonymous, 2001, p. 417). When you recognize this, you can begin to practice acceptance and attempt to turn the situation over to your Higher Power – trusting that He knows what is best. You pray that God's will be done and practice Step 11 by praying, "for knowledge of His will for us and the power to carry that out" (Alcoholics Anonymous, 2001, p. 59). This gets you out of your will and into God's will. The usual result is that you no longer have anything to be angry about.

The above anger management tools are very practical and really work in managing anger in most cases. You will also find that some tools, like exercise or inconspicuous yelling, are particularly effective when you are extremely angry. Using such tools allows you to calm down enough to utilize other tools like calling your sponsor, journaling, or praying so you can work through the anger.

More Anger Management Ideas

A major key to successful anger management is to catch it before you act it out negatively. All the anger management tools in the world are of no value if the anger is not recognized before you hurt yourself or others through one of your tantrums or by relapsing. Remember, you are dealing with your sobriety here. To over-react to your anger may be to drink or use and eventually die. So it is very important to learn to anticipate your anger and manage it as it comes. However, this is much easier said than done.

> So it is very important to learn to antici-pate your anger and manage it as it comes.

The key to training yourself to anticipate your anger is to make its management a high priority in your life. This is only done through the recognition that your anger will eventually lead you to relapse and you very much want to avoid that. Once you have made anger manage-ment a high priority in your life, you will take your anger management very seriously. Each time you begin to get angry, you will view it as a potential danger to your sobriety and quickly utilize your anger man-agement tools.

I have created an anger "acting out" continuum that will help you to catch your anger at increasingly earlier stages and intervene upon it be-fore it gets worse (see Figure 3 on page 124). This is a sample of what I have used in my own sobriety and you're invited to create one using your own examples of anger acting out. I have provided a template you can use to create this (Figure 4). First, write down many examples of unhealthy ways you act out on your anger. Now rank them in order of severity. Then place the most severe items toward the end of the continuum marked "10," followed by the next most severe items near the "9" and so forth. Note, on the example I have provided, that as you move toward the left end of the continuum, the acting out is much less severe. In fact, at number "1," you actually anticipate situations which make you angry and either avoid them, or create an anger management plan for dealing with the anger-provoking situation.

Application of this continuum can aid you in measuring how you are progressing in anticipating and dealing with your anger. Every time you have an angry episode, you check your continuum to see how far down the scale you have gone in your anger acting out. If you have gone further down the scale than you are comfortable with at a given stage in your development, you should commit yourself to trying to do better next time and pray that you might accomplish this. The uncomfortable feeling and fear of relapse you experience in falling short of your expectations can help drive you to do better the next time. If you see any improvement in the anticipation and management of your anger, give yourself some positive strokes and, perhaps, reward yourself. If you are consistent in gauging how you've done in such situations, you will notice a gradual improvement and find yourself more often toward the left end of the continuum. Remember, to succeed in this, use your fear of relapse as a driving force in making anger management a high priority – it is essential!

Figure 3

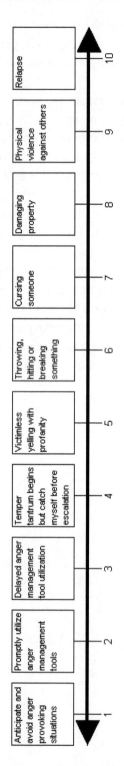

Anger "Acting-out" Continuum

1	Anticipate and avoid anger provoking situations
2	Promptly utilize anger management tools
3	Delayed anger management tool utilization
4	Temper tantrum begins but catch myself before escalation
5	Victimless yelling with profanity
6	Throwing, hitting or breaking something
7	Cursing someone
8	Damaging property
9	Physical violence against others
10	Relapse

Figure 4

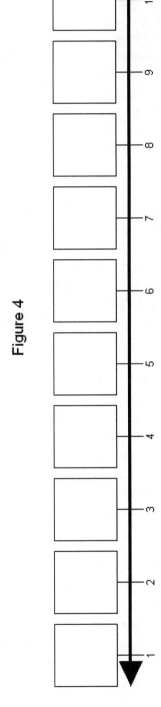

Anger "Acting-out" Continuum

Fear

Excessive fear is a trait that most alcoholics and addicts have. We seem to have more fear, of more things, than normal people do. Such fear totally encompasses us to the point that we often anesthetize it just as we do other uncomfortable feelings. The Big Book describes it well: "This short word (fear) somehow touches about every aspect of our lives. It was an evil and corroding thread; the fabric of our existence was shot through with it. It set in motion trains of circumstances which brought us misfortune we felt we didn't deserve" (Alcoholics Anonymous, 2001, p. 69).

An acronym for fear commonly used in the program is **F**alse **E**vidence **A**ppearing **R**eal. Although the meaning of this can be taken in many ways, I choose to believe that the false evidence is that which causes you to believe you have control over what happens in God's world. You fear that you lack control over things that might hurt yourself or others. Well guess what? You're right. You do lack that kind of power. And as soon as you accept this fact, you can surrender to a Higher Power who controls all:

> "Perhaps there is a better way – we think so. For we are now on a different basis; the basis of trusting and relying upon God. We trust infinite God rather than our finite selves. We are in the world to play the role He assigns. Just to the extent that we do as we think he would have us, and humbly rely on Him, does He enable us to match calamity with serenity. …We ask Him to remove our fear and direct our attention to what He would have us be. At once, we commence to outgrow fear" (Alcoholics Anonymous, 2001, p. 68).

In Chapter 6, I asserted that the key to recovery is found within Step 3. You have proven that you have no control over alcohol and/or drugs and, in Step 1, you come to grips with this fact. Out of desperation you identify a Higher Power that does have the power to control it. In Step 3, you make "a decision to turn our will and our lives over to God *as we understood Him*" (Alcoholics Anonymous, 2001, p. 59). You then set upon working the remaining steps to accomplish what you made a decision to do in Step 3. But this decision goes far beyond turning your using over to Him. You turn your whole life over to Him – including what you want. You attempt to accept God's will rather than exerting your own. To the extent that you are able to do this, your fear is lessened. After all, if you are working toward what God wants rather than what you want, what do you have to fear? What you fear is that your will, no matter how noble, will not be realized. Again, if you are focused on what God wants, and God controls all, what do you have to fear? If you continue to fear, you must be concerned about your own will – not God's. I know this seems rather simplistic, but this is the attitude we work toward in recovery and its practice eventually pays dividends in the form of serenity.

Grief and Loss

Along with shame and fear, grief is a very difficult feeling to experience. Life is full of losses. We lose people, possessions, and situations we enjoyed or valued, and even feel loss when we don't get what we want – even though we never had it in the first place. This is not just because we are alcoholics and drug addicts. Everyone loses these things. And, like the other emotions discussed above, grief is God-given. As uncomfortable as grief is, it is a healthy and normal process. Therefore, it should not be avoided – it should be felt just like all emotions.

As with the other emotions, alcoholics and addicts are very intolerant of grief. Since you have been covering up your grief with the use of substances, your first instinct when you experience grief is to run. When you make a commitment for sobriety, you often try to stuff down your grief in other ways, such as: ignoring it, engaging in other dysfunctional or compulsive behaviors, or masking it with other emotions. The key in recovery is to work your program tools so you can go through the *natural* process of grieving.

Five Stages of Grief

Dr. Elisabeth Kubler-Ross, (1969) identifies five stages of grief in her work with people with terminal illness:

- Denial
- Anger
- Sorrow/Despair/Depression
- Bargaining
- Acceptance

In his pamphlet, *Grieving: A Healing Process (1985)*, Peter Converse McDonald, M.Div., states, "Every stage of the process is natural and healthy (even denial!)" (p. 5). He also states that, "Although not a stage of the grieving process itself, fear underlies all other stages. We fear loss of control. We fear being what we think we'll be if we admit our dependency on alcohol or anything else. We fear powerlessness because we think if we're not in control, no one is! If we don't stay in control, we'll die!" (p. 5). Keep this fear of lack of control in mind as we review what McDonald has to say about the stages of grief. Remember, each of these stages is a natural and healthy part of the grieving process.

Denial

According to McDonald, "Denial is a psychological buffer that protects us from knowledge or feelings we're not yet ready to deal with mentally, emotionally, or spiritually. All of us deny reality we're not ready to accept" (p. 6). It is as if denial buys us some time so we can slowly begin to face the reality of the situation. The reality is that the situation did happen and we are powerless to do anything about it. When we begin to attain a mental understanding that the loss did happen, we then turn to anger regarding our powerlessness over the situation.

Anger

McDonald states that feeling angry with someone for dying, or feeling angry when we can't find something, are natural and healthy responses to loss (pp. 5-6). "It's exactly the same with chemical dependency or codependency. It just makes us furious that we can't control our own or someone else's behavior and feelings" (p. 7). Again, the anger you feel is due to loss of control, and the key to getting through it is the same as mentioned above – you accept your anger and work the tools of recovery as you experience it.

Sorrow/Despair/Depression

According to McDonald: "This is the response we normally associate with grief, but it's actually only one part of the whole process. Tears and sobbing are ways sorrow is expressed. It's the natural, healthy way to express the sorrow anyone feels after a loss" (p. 7). This is often difficult for men in our society because "Big boys don't cry." This is hogwash! God gave you this mechanism to use when you are sad. You don't need an audience when you do it, and if you are embarrassed doing it around other people, then do it alone. If you allow yourself to cry, you are finally allowing yourself to feel uncomfortable emotions instead of running from them. In my personal experience, crying is the best way to surrender to a very difficult situation that I have no control over. It is a release that leads to healing. If you allow this process to occur, you are moving toward the goal of accepting your loss. But first, many of us visit the bargaining stage of grief before we move toward such acceptance.

Bargaining

According to McDonald: "Bargaining is a desperate attempt to stay in control, to have things the way we want them. Trying to control our use is bargaining: 'If I have only one or two drinks, it'll prove I'm in control and therefore not powerless'" (p. 9). He also states that bargaining is natural and healthy and is a form of denial because it guards us against reality we're not ready for (p. 9).

In all of the above stages, although they are healthy, McDonald warns that getting stuck in any of them can be destructive because it can eventually lead to destructive behavior (p. 6-10). Again, this is an issue of powerlessness. Bargaining, like the other stages, is a stepping-stone to the acceptance of our powerlessness.

Acceptance

McDonald states that the goal of the grieving process is acceptance:

> "...we come to accept the loss which has occurred. We accept that we are powerless over alcohol (or another substance or person), that we are not the people we thought we were. Having grieved, we can accept the loss of our power and go on with the rest of our lives, which is what the Twelve Steps are all about. Having grieved and accepted our powerlessness, we find serenity and peace. We have come to terms with reality" (p. 10).

Acceptance is the destination in the grieving process and it results from knowledge of the fact that you are utterly powerless over the situation and can't do anything about it. The 12-Step philosophy of turning it over to your Higher Power applies here as well. Due to your humanity limiting your ability to understand everything, you have to trust God with what he decides to do in His world. After all, there's nothing you can do about it anyway. This does not mean you have to like what happens in God's world – it only means you need to accept it and ask God to aid you in doing so.

I want to take a moment here to address the significance of having to lose your drug of choice. One might think that, since drugs and alcohol have done so much damage in your life, you should be happy to give them up. I don't know about you, but I was not happy at all. For most of us, it is like giving up a best friend – something that we could always count on to take away the pain. It was with us through thick and thin. It was the one thing we could do to escape our seemingly constant pain. Regarding our drug of choice, most of us enjoyed using it, at least temporarily. I could not pretend that I just did not like doing it anymore despite all the damage it caused in my life.

You might find this kind of strange coming from someone who has nearly 25 years of sobriety and who has dedicated his life to helping others attain it, but if I didn't have consequences associated with using, I would love nothing better than to take a big hit of cocaine. However, I do have consequences and I am not willing to face them today. I have proven beyond a shadow of a doubt that I can never again safely use any mind-altering substance. Therefore, despite how much I enjoyed using them, I had to grieve losing drugs and alcohol. I strongly believe that this is a very important part of recovery.

One way to tap into such grief is to write a good-bye letter to your drug of choice. I wish I still had the letter I wrote so I could share it with you. However, my sponsor recommended that, after reading it to him, I should burn it as a gesture of closure. I will, however, share with you what the letter sounded like to the best of my recollection:

Dear Candy,

As difficult as it is for me to do this, I have to say good-bye to you. This hurts me very much because we had many good times together. I loved when we got together with friends and got smashed. We didn't have a care in the world and I loved the camaraderie we had with our using buddies. You also helped me very much in difficult times. You comforted me like no one else could and you were always there when I needed you. It saddens and scares me very much to let you go.

However, somewhere along the line you turned on me you bitch! You cost me my integrity; you made me go against nearly every moral I ever had; you almost cost me my job; and you made me hurt my wife to the point she had to leave. I hate you for this and I never want to see you again!

My wife and I are back together now and I'll be damned if I'm going to let you get in our way. I don't ever want you to present your ugly head to me again. Knowing how devious you are, I'm sure you'll try to make your way back into my life like you have so many times before. But it will not work this time because I have realized that I am powerless against your advances alone. I now have a relationship with God who is much stronger and wiser than to fall for your tricks and I will gladly step aside so God can kick your ass if you get near me. Goodbye and good riddance. I can't wait to see how good my life is going to get without you!

Sincerely,
Bob

Wow! Just taking myself through that exercise again brought up a lot of feelings. I can remember how emotional I was while originally writing that letter. I highly recommend you write such a letter as a beginning toward getting on with your life.

I must also mention here the grief I felt having to give up the friends and acquaintances that would get in the way of my recovery if I continued seeing them. This was very difficult for me as I very much valued the people in my life. However, I must admit to you that most of the people I am talking about were more using buddies than they were friends. Without the one major thing we had in common – our love for drugs and alcohol – there was very little left to base a relationship upon. At the time I was first getting sober, it was difficult for me to see this.

I also needed to grieve the lifestyle that was part of my alcohol and drug use. I used to love getting together with the guys, going to a sporting event, and getting hammered with them. Again, I could not pretend this was something I didn't desire anymore. It was something I loved but needed to give it up. Therefore, this was something I also needed to grieve. Sobriety is not about doing the things I want to do – it is about doing what I have to do. Sobriety often takes sacrifice, but such sacrifice has paid dividends in my recovery. Now I *want* to be sober.

Along these same lines, when I was about six months sober, I decided to take my first weeklong vacation in sobriety. As I was contemplating this vacation, it suddenly occurred to me that I was not going to be able to use drugs or alcohol. It scared the heck out of me and saddened me deeply. In fantasizing about past vacations, I would see myself sitting on my ski boat on the Colorado river with a beer in one hand, a joint in the other, and cocaine waiting for me back at camp. I would gladly work 51 weeks out of the year to have this one week of doing what I enjoyed most. So when I discussed this issue of not using on my vacation, I became very emotional and began grieving it right there in group. I received much support and empathy from the group members. Many could really relate to my grieving. As it turns out, my wife and I had a great sober time in the Bahamas. It was one of the best vacations I ever had – and I remember it!

Finally, I will wrap up this section on grief with some suggestions by McDonald which aid in the grieving process (pp 11-14):

- Feel the feelings
- Allow yourself to cry
- Talk to someone
- Allow your anger
- Get into action – do something
- Write a good-bye letter
- Sing or whistle
- Laugh
- Pray and meditate
- Work the First Step
- New activities and friends

Note the overlap between these aids to grieving and the ingredients for recovery. This stuff really works, but it takes getting on your feet and participating in your recovery.

We have discussed above some of the difficult feelings that are simply a part of everyday life. We alcoholics and addicts are very intolerant of such feelings and we need to begin making it okay to feel. This is a major key to your recovery because the purpose of your drug use was to mask such feelings. If you can become tolerant, or even comfortable with feeling emotion, you will no longer have a reason to use drugs. I wish I could exhibit for you how fulfilling life is being able to feel the natural human emotion associated with living life on life's terms. My quality of life has exceeded my wildest dreams and expectations. My wish for you is that you get to have this experience. I realize that this takes a level of trust in some guy in recovery who wrote a book. But don't just take my word for it – look around. There are thousands of recovering alcoholics and addicts who can sincerely make you the same promise. So quit trusting what you think and begin trusting others – you won't regret it.

> If you can become tolerant, or even comfortable with feeling emotion, you will no longer have a reason to use drugs.

CHAPTER 8
STRUCTURING RECOVERY INTO YOUR DAILY LIVING

To give yourself the best chance at success in recovery, you will need to incorporate recovery into your daily living. I recommend starting your day ten or fifteen minutes earlier than normal to spend some time focused on your recovery first thing in the morning. As mentioned earlier, you might start by reading the daily passage from your morning meditation book. If you have already developed some concept of a Higher Power, you might follow your reading with a prayer that includes a request that you stay sober that day. If you have not yet developed a concept of a Higher Power, go ahead and go through the motions anyway – you may be surprised at the impact it has on you.

As soon as possible, make a copy of the master list of the "ingredients for recovery," "triggers," and "warning signs." Remember to highlight items on the latter two lists that you think apply particularly to you. After your Morning Prayer, view all three of these lists so they are fresh on your mind as you start your day.

Next, think over what you have planned for that particular day and evaluate whether or not any of these plans might be dangerous to your recovery. If anything you have planned for that day could be a trigger to relapse, change or alter your plans accordingly. Remember, it is essential in early recovery to avoid any drinking/using situations, or people who drink or use. Later in your recovery you will be able to gradually re-introduce some such drinking situations back into your life, but now is not the time. Also, it is essential to safely remove all alcohol, drugs, and paraphernalia from your home to eliminate such triggers. Elimination of these items makes drinking and using less convenient. If you consider leaving such items in your house, you are probably leaving them there so you can use again.

> Remember, down time will allow your mind to drift to where it wants to go, and it will most assuredly go places it doesn't belong.

Review your plans each day to determine if there is any down time and plan to fill such time by doing something constructive that will keep you busy. Remember, down time will allow your mind to drift to where it wants to go, and it will most assuredly go places it doesn't belong. If you don't currently have much structure in your day, you might consider a job, school, volunteer work, or a healthy hobby that will keep you occupied much of the day. I strongly recommend going to multiple meetings during the day until you have incorporated such structure. Many people start their day with an early morning or noon meeting to break up their day with recovery.

Begin reading the Big Book (or the textbook of your program of choice) on a daily basis. You might do this in the evening before you go to bed or simply when you have some free time. I have found it helpful to read some of the book in the evening followed by some evening prayer that includes gratitude for my sobriety that day.

Once you get a sponsor and establish your powerlessness and unmanageability by working Step 1, I recommend writing your good-bye letter. Also keep in mind as you work the steps, your sponsor is likely having you work the steps as he or she worked them. Follow his or her direction regarding the steps and other elements in your recovery. Remember, you chose your sponsor because you want what he or she has. If you do what your sponsor did in recovery, you will likely receive the gifts that attracted you to your sponsor. If a suggestion from your sponsor seems outlandish to you, simply ask other members of the fellowship who have significant sober time if they agree with the suggestion. If it appears from your inquiry that the request is unreasonable, simply tell your sponsor your concerns and that you are not willing to follow such direction. If your sponsor still insists, you may need to find another sponsor. I give you these suggestions regarding sponsor direction, not to get you focused on questioning your sponsor's suggestions, but to encourage you to protect yourself against potentially damaging advice. This is clearly the exception rather than the rule.

Given that you have probably been holding your feelings at bay for some time, you will now have to learn to feel such feelings without drugs and alcohol. I firmly believe that the key to staying off of drugs and alcohol is the ability to tolerate emotion as it arises. There are at least three very important factors involved in dealing with such emotion. First, a sober support system is essential. You have proven that you are incapable of tolerating emotion on your own. You must bring others into it. When you experience uncomfortable emotions, you need to talk the feelings through with others who understand how difficult emotion is for alcoholics and addicts to experience. What you are accomplishing by talking the feelings through is that you are fully experiencing the emotion, rather than running from it, with the support of another recovering alcoholic or addict.

> I firmly believe that the key to staying off of drugs and alcohol is the ability to tolerate emotion as it arises.

Next, you also need to come to believe in a Higher Power that you can trust to help you through such difficult times. The path of recovery, as outlined in the 12-Steps, guides you toward a surrender that enables you to allow God to control what happens in the world. This gives you the comfort of knowing that all you are responsible for is the footwork towards His will and that He will take care of the rest. If you are truly able to accomplish this, there is no longer anything to worry about. Remember, this is a process. I'm not sure this is ever fully accomplished, but the level at which you are able to achieve this will increase the longer you are working your program.

Finally, you need to make it okay to feel lousy once in a while. As mentioned earlier, our first reaction when we get an emotion is typically, "Run!" A better reaction is, "Boy, does this feel lousy. However, emotion is natural and I need to get some support while I am experiencing this." A good program saying that helps during such times is: *"This, too, shall pass."* Besides, you must experi-

> ...you need to make it okay to feel lousy once in a while.

ence highs and lows so life doesn't become boring and monotonous. Remember, to feel emotion is to be fully human.

Pay special attention to how you react to emotions – especially anger. Most of us have not reacted well to our anger in the past. This often results in negative consequences and embarrassment. Although you won't achieve perfection in controlling your anger, you need to constantly strive to improve how you react to it. This is done by working the elements of recovery described above – bringing others into it, working your spiritual program, and making it okay to be angry once in a while without having to react to it in a way that prevents you from working through it.

In living a life of recovery, keeping sobriety as the number one priority is essential. If sobriety is truly number one, everything that you have done or plan to do each day, needs to be scrutinized as it relates to your chances for long-term sobriety. This is why it is so important to start each day by reviewing your plans to ensure that your sobriety will not be endangered. The same is true for when you end your day. Reflect on the day that has passed to analyze how you have put your sobriety at risk and learn from it. This will be done more formally when you get to Step 10, but I recommend doing it now to enhance your chances at making it to that step. Remember, if sobriety is truly number one, every decision that you make during the course of your day should be made keeping potential relapse in mind.

A counselor I worked with at St. John's in Santa Monica, often used to encourage her patients to ask themselves at any given stage in their recovery, "Are you on the road to relapse or on the road to recovery?" The question was to be asked as if there was no in-between – you were on one of two paths. I encourage you to ask yourself this question on a regular basis. If you have any question about which road you are on, get into action immediately, utilizing the tools for recovery. Be persistent until you can honestly say to yourself that you are on the road to recovery.

Whatever you do, *don't get cocky.* This disease is more powerful than you are and as soon as you think you have it licked and get complacent, it will jump up and bite you just as it has so many

> Whatever you do, *don't get cocky.*

times before. Always remember when you first started this trek into recovery and were whipped by your addiction. You may have bought this book out of desperation and you probably didn't know the first thing about recovery. Don't make the mistake of some of your predecessors and suddenly think you know what is best for you. Always seek out feedback from your sponsor, and sober peers, whenever there is a significant decision to be made – especially if it has to do with your program of recovery. Never think you have all the answers and that you don't need the program anymore. The level of humility you retain will directly correlate with your chances at long-term sobriety.

Recovery is a lot of work, but the results are absolutely worth it. Be persistent and continue to work a strong recovery program so you can keep the gifts you acquire, and to make yourself available for further miracles.

CHAPTER 9
THE MIRACLE

In the introduction to this book, I mentioned a man by the name of Jim Fulton whom I was very angry at for telling my wife not to talk to me in my early treatment. After all, I was getting help for my problem and who was he to dictate when my wife and I should talk? Little did I know, Jim would turn out to be the most skilled counselor and caring man I have ever known. He had an uncanny ability to understand what was happening inside of me and to explain it in terms I could understand. Jim was also able to help me identify the true source of my feelings and help me work through them.

In Chapter 7, I wrote about the time my dad predicted that all of my brothers would have respectable jobs and that I would become a trash collector. I carried much resentment about this incident as I felt it contributed greatly to my low self-esteem. In a group session, after allowing me to process and feel my anger, Jim suggested the possibility that I could paint myself a better picture about what happened that day. The picture I had painted about that situation is that Dad really felt that way about me. After all, I didn't recall being in trouble about anything that day. Consequently, since he was my male role model and someone whose feedback I took seriously, I felt that I really must be worthless.

Jim suggested there might be other ways I could look at that situation. With his help, I was able to paint myself a better picture about what happened. The new picture I painted suggested that I may not have been doing well in school at the time and, since Dad cared about me, was trying to motivate me the best way he knew how. Although I believe the negative impact of his intervention outweighed the positive, this new scenario suggests he meant well. Now, this possibility may not have been true, but if I am really honest with myself, it is more likely true than the picture I previously painted about the situation. As a result of this, and working the 12-Step program (especially Step 4), I have rid myself of the resentment toward my father and we have a good relationship today. Coming from where I was in that situation, this is truly a miracle in my life.

I would like to add here that it was the skill of Jim Fulton that attracted me to this profession. By the time I left treatment, I was convinced that becoming a counselor was for me, and others were giving me feedback that I would be a good one. At nine months sober, I decided to go back to school to learn how to become a counselor. Ten years prior, despite the fact that I did not earn enough units to get a high school diploma, I was allowed to participate in my graduation ceremony since I was within fifteen units of the graduation requirements (in the midst of my addiction, I skipped school frequently to get loaded). I then procrastinated for seven years before I finally achieved enough adult school units to get my diploma. However, when I presented my high school with the necessary units, I was told the requirements had gone up and that I needed another year of English and math to get it. I wasn't willing to do that so I gave up on the idea of getting a high school diploma.

Mary Catherine Fitzgerald, my family counselor, who was largely responsible for Robin and me working things out and getting back together, was also the director of the Alcohol and Drug Studies Program at Loyola Marymount University (LMU). She told me that if I wanted to get into the program at LMU, I would need a high school diploma or pass the GED test. She also told me I might be able to get a scholarship for the program there. With this information, I set out to reach my goal.

Since I wanted to get into the college as soon as possible, I took the GED test and passed. The next step was to obtain my high school transcripts. Now this was scary. I had not done well in high school, as I was too busy getting loaded. I received my transcripts and found that I had a 1.3 grade point average (just better than a "D"). If that wasn't bad enough, I also found out that I was ranked 392nd out of 392 students – dead last! Boy, that was a rude awakening!

I succeeded in not only getting into LMU, but also in receiving a scholarship (probably both resulting from Mary Catherine pulling some strings). I was really feeling God's work in my life! I ended up doing very well in the Alcohol and Drug Studies Program and eventually went back to school to get a degree in psychology. I graduated with honors and a 3.97 grade point average. Another miracle of the program!

Shortly after I started at LMU, Jim was hired as the Program Director at the very prestigious chemical dependence program at St. John's Hospital in Santa Monica. It was as if God rolled out the red carpet for me as soon as I made the decision to become a counselor. Naturally, I did my internship there and was eventually hired by Jim.

Jim had become my mentor and I truly loved him. He was responsible for helping me turn my life around and also for leading me into a career that is very spiritually rewarding. After about a year at St. John's, I noticed that Jim was sick a lot and was losing weight rapidly. I confronted him about this as I felt he was being evasive as to what was wrong with him. My worst fear was realized as he told me he had a terminal illness. I was devastated. I didn't know how I would survive watching my beloved friend and mentor die. In my early recovery, I had this sick fantasy that if a tragedy happened in my life, I would have an excuse to use. This certainly fell into that category.

Jim deteriorated quickly and eventually moved to Kentucky to be with his mother. I got word that he was close to death so I made the trip to Kentucky to say good-bye. As I said good-bye, I kissed him on the forehead and promised I would continue his work to the best of my ability. I left and walked to the parking lot at the VA and wept for hours. I boarded a plane home and, three weeks later, I received word that he had died. As much pain as I was in through that whole process, it never occurred to me to get loaded – still another miracle of the program!

On the other end of the continuum of life, Robin and I had been trying to have children for three years prior to my getting sober. I remember in my early recovery shedding tears at meetings over this and wondering if I would ever be a father. Part of me believed God didn't feel I was ready yet to have children. Two years into my sobriety, we decided to get more aggressive about it and started infertility treatment. However, five months passed and Robin still wasn't pregnant.

Finally, a couple months after a very relaxing (and intimate) trip to Aspen, Colorado, it happened. I'll never forget the feeling I had when Robin told me she was pregnant. It was pure elation. I was very aware that this, again, was God working in our lives. I also took it as a compliment from God that He felt I was ready. We now have four children and they are the joys of my life – pure gifts of sobriety.

One of the true pleasures of working in the profession of chemical dependency is getting to see the miracles of sobriety on a daily basis. At Twin Town Treatment Centers, where I oversee program operations at six different locations, we treat approximately 50 – 60 new patients per month. As you might imagine with this type of volume, we see the miracle of sobriety all the time. I am still amazed when it happens and it never gets old. I could write a separate book based on such miracles, but I will briefly describe only one here.

It happened when I was working at St. John's toward the beginning of my career. A very sick man entered detox because his drinking had done irreparable damage to his liver and to one of his kidneys. He would not be considered a candidate for transplants unless he quit drinking. This man was a high level executive of a multi-million dollar company. You would never know it by looking at him. He was yellow in color and his abdomen was extremely swollen from the organ damage. He was a pleasant man and it was very painful to look at him. Amazingly, he was still in a lot of denial about his disease. As I attempted to help him break through his denial, I felt as if I was speaking to a dead man. In no way did I believe he could survive. After some success in helping him break through his denial, he was discharged and I was sure he would die soon and I would never see him again.

About a year passed when a good-looking man, whom I did not recognize, approached the nurse's station where I was working. I greeted him and asked how I could help him. When he identified himself as that same man, I almost hit the floor. He explained that he had re-

mained sober ever since he had visited our unit and that he had received successful liver and kidney transplants. He was back to work at
the corporation and his life had been given back to him. The elation I
experienced by seeing this amazing transformation had my eyes well-
ing up with tears. If you think that your life is beyond divine intervention, I hope such a story gives you some hope.

As I wrote earlier, I believe spirituality is simply an awareness of the
presence of a Higher Power. Since I try to live a spiritual life, I am often aware of God's presence and his work in my life. What I used to
write off as neat coincidences, are now seen as God's divine interventions. There is one more such intervention that I would like to share
with you. You can judge for yourself whether you feel a Higher Power
is working in my life – I am convinced of it.

It happened when I was about nine months sober. Robin and I had
gone on a seven-day trip to Great Abaco Island in the Bahamas. I had
assumed AA meetings would be available, but there were none on the
island. Fortunately, I brought a Big Book with me so I could stay
somewhat centered in my program. When we returned from the trip, I
hadn't attended a meeting for a whole week and decided I better go to
one that night. However, I got word that Stevie Ray Vaughn was playing the final concert of his local tour that night. Stevie Ray had been
my favorite musical artist so my decision was very difficult. Up to that
point in my sobriety, I usually made a decision that would be best for
my sobriety. Having not attended a meeting in a week, I was not
pumping on all cylinders program-wise and decided to attend the concert.

Robin and I arrived a little early to the show at the Greek Amphithea-
tre. We took our seats and participated in one our favorite past-times –
people-watching. We were there for a short while when two guys sitting to my right began smoking a joint. I was a connoisseur of marijuana and this was top-quality stuff. We used to call it "skunk-bud" (it is
now called "chronic"). Boy, did it smell good! Almost immediately
afterward, the couple sitting to the left of my wife fired up and it also
smelled like skunk-bud. I suddenly felt myself weakening and even
beginning to think about how I might sneak a hit without Robin notic-
ing. It was a very uncomfortable feeling as sobriety was of ultimate

importance to me. However, I had passed into the craving cycle, which causes addicts like me to have distorted thinking. Just as the rationalizations for use began to creep in, my eyes suddenly fell upon a welcome sight.

We were sitting way in the back of the outdoor arena, about fifty yards from the entrance, which was just left of the stage. I don't know why I happened to be looking that far away, but I noticed a man enter the arena who was wearing a shirt with a large circle-triangle (the AA insignia) on the front. My attention shifted immediately off the possibility of relapse and onto this man as he made his way up the stairs to the center aisle. I watched as he walked across the center aisle, started up the stairs right toward where we were sitting, turned down the row right in front of us, and sat in the seat directly in front of me! My eyes rose to the sky in acknowledgement of God as I recognized he was once again working in my life. I promptly tapped the man on the shoulder and we had our own little meeting right there. I told him what was happening and we both marveled at this divine intervention. If that wasn't enough, right before the concert was ready to start, a couple walked down the row right in front of us, tapped the same gentleman on the shoulder and informed him he was sitting in the wrong seat – he was about four rows off! I was feeling very spiritual then, and, when Stevie Ray started into his southern blues routine, I was thoroughly enjoying myself.

The divine intervention was not over. Stevie Ray started playing a song and, as he usually did when playing that particular song, stopped playing in order to address the audience while his band played lightly in the background. I usually enjoyed what he had to say during this song, but this time my enjoyment was magnified ten-fold. It went something like this, "I want to thank God for lettin' me be here with y'all tonight because I almost didn't make it this far. Ya know, nobody ever told me that when I went to a party, I had to go home some day. But the first thing I had to do was admit I had a problem with drugs and alcohol so I could git help. So y'all be careful out there 'cause alcohol and drugs can take ya down." He was 12th-Stepping the whole audience! Needless to say, I was standing and yelling at the top of my lungs during his pitch and the guy that God sent to me in my moment of need was doing the same. I felt very validated that this person, whom I had idolized, truly understood and had gone through the same nightmarish type of life that I had and that he, too, had received a second chance.

My wish for you is that you have a divine intervention in your life that will give you a second chance. Maybe picking up this book can be the start of your miracle. I hope the information I have shared helps you to understand that you're not alone and there is help for you if you are willing to receive it. All you need to do is get yourself out of the way of the miracle. If you can follow the direction of those before you who have found the path of recovery, you will experience the same miracle we have. You now have the information you need to begin getting your life back. Now it is up to you to go after it. In closing, I will quote the end of the chapter in the Big Book entitled *A Vision for You,* "...you will surely meet some of us as you trudge the Road of Happy Destiny. May God bless you and keep you – until then (Alcoholics Anonymous, 2001, p. 164)."

For sober coaching and/or online recovery counseling/educational opportunities with Bob Tyler, please visit his website at www.bobtyler.net and hit the "Sober Coaching" tab at the top of the page.

APPENDIX 1

Since the original publishing of this book, I have stumbled upon an incredibly effective recovery tool: "Mass Texting"©. Here's how it works:

First, get phone numbers from people you meet at your 12 Step meetings who will represent your sober support system (at least 20.) Enter the numbers into your cell phone and place a "code," i.e., a number (1, 2, 3, etc.), or letter, (x, y, z, etc.) in front of the contact's name so that all of your recovery numbers are grouped together in your phone's directory for easy access.

Mass Texting is used when you are in some sort of crisis, i.e., you feel like drinking or using, feel angry, fearful, sad or experiencing any other emotion. You simply send a text to multiple members of your support system letting them know you need to connect. With my phone, which is a quite old (not an iPhone), I can text up to 20 people at a time. The text might go something like this: "Hey guys, I was just triggered because I saw someone smoking a joint. I don't think I'm going to use, but was really triggered and felt I should call it out."

Without fail, the response is similar to this: at least one or two of my guys will call me back right away; about six to eight guys will send a supportive text and possibly let me know I can call if I need to (which in itself is very comforting); and those who can't get back to me right away text and call throughout the day to see how I'm doing. So, in effect, I have just bought myself a day full of contact with my sober support system with one simple action. It is a great tool and I highly recommend it!

APPENDIX 2

Alcoholics Anonymous (AA) World Services - (212) 870-3400
www.aa.org

Narcotics Anonymous (NA) World Services - (818) 773-9999
www.na.org

Cocaine Anonymous (CA) World Services - (310) 559-5833
www.ca.org

Crystal Meth Anonymous (CMA) (855) 638-4373
www.crystalmeth.org

Marijuana Anonymous World Services - (800) 766-6779
www.marijuana-anonymous.org

Pills Anonymous World Services - (800) 321-2211
www.pillsanonymous.org

Al-Anon Family Group Headquarters - (757) 563-1600
www.al-anon.alateen.org

Adult Children of Alcoholics (ACA) World Services - (562) 595-7831
www.adultchildren.org

National Suicide Prevention Lifeline - (800) 273-TALK (8255)

Treatment Referral Line - (800) 662-HELP (4357)
http://findtreatment.samhsa.gov/

Find a doctor:
http://www.freemedicalsearch.org/

Find a therapist, psychiatrist, therapy group, or treatment center:
www.PsychologyToday.com

APPENDIX 3

Meeting Verification Card

Name:		
Date	Meeting Name	Secretary Signature

Permission to copy this page for personal use is granted.

REFERENCES

Alcoholics Anonymous World Services, Inc. (2001). *Alcoholics Anonymous*. 4th ed. New York: Alcoholics Anonymous World Services, Inc.

Gorski, Terence T. (Speaker). (1988). *Cocaine craving and relapse: A comparison between alcohol and cocaine* (Cassette Recording No. 17 – 0157). Independence, Mo: Herald House/Independence Press.

Gorski, Terence T. (1989, April). Cocaine craving and relapse. *Sober Times: The Recovery Magazine,* 3 (4), pp. 6, 29.

Gorski, Terence T. (2001). *Cocaine, craving, and relapse.* [On-line]. Available Internet: http://www.tgorski.com/gorski_articles/co caine%20craving%20&%20relapse%20010523.htm.

Gorski, Terence T., and Merlene Miller. (1986). *Staying Sober: A Guide for Relapse Prevention.* Independence, Mo: Herald House/Independence Press.

Johnson, Helen M. (1986). *How Do I Love Me?* Salem, WI: Sheffield Publishing Company.

Kinney, Jean, and Gwen Leaton. (1987). *Loosening the Grip.* 3rd ed. St. Louis: Times Mirror/Mosby Company.

Kubler-Ross, Elisabeth. (1969). *On Death and Dying.* New York: Macmillan Publishing Co., Inc.

McDonald, Peter Converse. (1985) *Grieving: A healing process.* Minneapolis, MN: Hazelden Publications.

McKechnie, Jean L. (1983). *Webster's New Twentieth Century Dictionary of the English Language Unabridged.* 2nd ed. New York: Simon and Schuster.

Pagewise, Inc. (2002). *This study in classical conditioning is one of the most renown for its incredible results. Learn about Pav-Dogs!* [On-line]. Available Internet: http://ks.essortment.com/ Pavlovdogs_oif.htm.

Wanigaratne, Shamil, et al. (1990). *Relapse Prevention for Addictive Behaviors. Oxford: Blackwell Scientific Pubications*

ABOUT THE AUTHOR

Bob Tyler, BA, CADC II, ICADC has been working in the chemical dependence recovery field since 1990. After beginning his personal recovery from alcohol and drug addiction in December of 1988, he completed the Alcohol and Drug Studies Program at Loyola Marymount University (LMU) and graduated *Summa Cum Laude* with a Bachelor of Arts Degree in Psychology at LMU. As of the printing of this edition, Bob is the Director of Operations and Clinical Services for Twin Town Treatment Centers where he is responsible for six intensive outpatient treatment locations – each serving the chemical dependence treatment needs of adults and adolescents.

Bob is certified by the California Association of Alcohol and Drug Abuse Counselors (CAADAC) and by the International Certification and Reciprocity Consortium (ICRC). Beginning in 1997, he served on the Board of Directors of CAADAC for fourteen years, chairing the Quality Assurance and Third Party/Managed Care Committees until becoming President-Elect in 2005. Bob served as CAADAC President from 2007 – 2009. He is currently the Treasurer of the California Foundation for the Advancement of Addiction Professionals (CFAAP).

Bob serves on the Advisory Boards for Alcohol and Drug Studies Programs at multiple colleges and universities across Southern California. As of this printing, he is also a member of the faculty at LMU Extension in the Alcohol and Drug Studies Program.

It is Bob's vision that this book and its contents be utilized to aid those who suffer from the diseases of alcoholism and other drug addiction. He is hopeful that it directly reaches alcoholics and addicts, students who aspire to become addiction counselors, and counselors in or out of treatment centers who treat addictions.

www.bobtyler.net

CPSIA information can be obtained
at www.ICGtesting.com
Printed in the USA
FSHW04n2318220418
47281FS

9 781598 002133